ALAN R. STOCKARD, D.O., FAOASM

Osteopathic Clinical Joint Exam

American Osteopathic Academy of Sports Medicine
2424 American Lane
Madison WI 53704-3102

Production Editor: Amy Bayer
Cover Design: The Rees Group, Inc.
Typesetter: Cynthia Coates
Printed by: Documation, LLC
Printed in the United States of America.

10 9 8 7 6 5 4 3 2 1

American Osteopathic Academy of Sports Medicine
2424 American Lane
Madison WI 53704-3102
608.443.2477 (phone)
608.443.2474 (fax)
www.aoasm.org (web)

Table of Contents

Page
Number

PREFACE

During the past 20 years of teaching as full-time faculty at two Colleges of Osteopathic Medicine, as well as precepting Osteopathic Medical students from all over the country in clinical rotations, I have noticed a common trend. Graduates of our Colleges of Osteopathic Medicine (COMs) have a very limited knowledge of the basic orthopedic/ osteopathic joint exam. While many are capable of performing an adequate Osteopathic musculoskeletal assessment, and others can perform a rudimentary orthopedic exam, very few are able to "put it all together" into one seamless examination. A study that Thomas Allen, D.O., and I published in 2006 documented that graduates of COMs do not have significantly superior joint exam skills or knowledge than graduates of allopathic schools.

Osteopathic Clinical Joint Exam is intended to present a comprehensive approach to musculoskeletal complaints by detailing the basic exam using both osteopathic and orthopedic techniques in a concise way with the goal of arriving at a differential diagnosis based on (history and) clinical exam alone. This was the type of medicine practiced by our Osteopathic forefathers before the advent of sophisticated diagnostic modalities such as Computerized Tomography, Magnetic Resonance Imaging, or ultrasound, and physicians became excellent clinicians as a result.

In today's medical and political climate, attempts at controlling medical costs are applauded, but the real winners are the patients who receive a good, thorough physical examination by a competent Osteopathic physician. Treatment options come more immediately to mind when certain conditions are ruled in or out based on the office exam, thereby drastically curtailing the need for costly diagnostic procedures. The sooner treatment begins without the delays of further testing, the sooner the patient benefits.

The contributing authors were specifically chosen due to their years of involvement in Osteopathic medical education and sports medicine, and because of the dedication to teaching that burns inside each of them. My hat is off to them for their incredible efforts, and my life is enhanced by being able to call them friends, as well as sports medicine colleagues. God bless you all!

This book owes a debt of gratitude to the monumental work of Steven Karageanes, D.O., who created the finest sports medicine reference book for Osteopathic physicians to date, *The Principles of Manual Sports Medicine* (Lippincott Williams & Wilkins, 2005). He graciously allowed us to use photos from his textbook for this manaul. Dr. Karageanes has shared his time and resources with us, and we are very grateful for his generosity. His book covers practically the entire spectrum of the practice of sports medicine and is an excellent stand-alone textbook. This volume is intended to distill only the important elements of the examination of the joints for the medical student or clinician. Thank you, Steve.

This text outlines the basic anatomy (a good refresher is always helpful), and the exam itself, followed by a list of the common conditions seen in clinical practice, and finally, by a list of conditions that should never be missed due to an incomplete exam. This will give the medical student, resident, or practicing physician a basis for decision-making, as well as a handbook that will, hopefully, provide invaluable information to all clinicians who encounter patients with musculoskeletal complaints.

Treatments and diagnostic tests are intentionally omitted as this is a text devoted exclusively to physical diagnosis. New and improved diagnostic modalities and even treatment options may come and go, but a good, thorough physical exam will always endure in medicine, and should never be supplanted by a machine.

Special thanks to Amy Bayer for her hours of diligent work in preparing this manuscript.

A.R.S.

AUTHOR BIOGRAPHIES

Thomas W. Allen, D.O., MPH
Clinical Professor of Family and Sports Medicine
University of Oklahoma
School of Community Medicine, TulsaVice President and Professor of Medicine Emeritus
Oklahoma State University Center for HealthSciences
Team Physician, Oklahoma State University Wrestling

Anna Avik, D.O., ATC
Orthopaedic Surgery Resident
Riverside County Regional Medical Center
Riverside, CA

Gregory C. Beato, D.O.
Medical Associates of Southwest Virginia
Blacksburg, VA
Team Physician, Virginia Tech and Floyd County High School

Fred H. Brennan, Jr., D.O., FAOASM, FAAFP, FACSM
Head Team Physician
University of New Hampshire
Medical Director
Seacoast Center for Athletes
Somersworth, New Hampshire

P. Gunnar Brolinson, D.O., FAOASM, FACOFP, FAAFP
Associate Dean for Clinical Research
Director, Primary Care Sports Medicine Fellowship
Virginia College of Osteopathic Medicine
Team Physician, Virginia Tech and US Ski Team

Stephen M. Daquino, D.O., FAOASM
Assistant Professor
Department of Family Medicine
New York College of Osteopathic Medicine
Team Physician, New York Institute of Technology & CW Post/Long Island University
Director, Primary Care Sports Medicine Fellowship at North Shore/LIJ Plainview Hospital

Douglas P. Dietzel, D.O.
Head Team Orthopedic Surgeon
Michigan State University
Associate Professor
Division of Orthopedics
College of Osteopathic Medicine
Clinical Director, MSU Sports Medicine
Orthopedic Residency Director - IRMC/MSU

John J. Dougherty, D.O., FAOASM
Professor of Family and Sports Medicine
Associate Dean of Clinical Education and Medical Affairs
Kansas City University of Medicine and Biosciences
Kansas City, MO

William M. Falls, Ph.D.
Associate Dean/Student Services
Professor of Anatomy
Department of Radiology
Division of Human Anatomy and Structural Biology
Michigan State University
College of Osteopathic Medicine
East Lansing, MI

R. Robert Franks, D.O., FAOASM
Assistant Director Sports Medicine
Director of Sports Concussion Program
Cooper Bone and Joint Institute
Cooper University Hospital
Voorhees, NJ
Assistant Professor, Orthopedic Surgery, UMDNJ-RWJ
Clinical Assistant Professor of Family Medicine, UMDNJ-SOM, UMDNJ-RWJ
Team Physician, USA Wrestling, Philadelphia Wings Lacrosse

Kimberly Grillo, D.O.
Orthopedic Surgery Resident
Pontiac Osteopathic Hospital
Pontiac, MI

Michael Henehan, D.O., FAOASM
Past President, AOASM
Adjunct Clinical Professor in Family Medicine
Stanford University
Director, Sports Medicine Program at O'Connor Hospital
Team Physician, San Jose State University and San Jose Earthquakes Soccer Team

Shawn Kerger, D.O., CAQSM
Physician Education Specialist, Doctors Hospital
Associate Professor, Doctors Hospital Family Practice Residency
Columbus, OH

Bernard F. King, D.O., FAOASM, FAAFP
Past President, AOASM
Private Practice
Wilmington, DE

Kathryn C. Lambert, D.O., CAQSM
Assistant Dean for Student Affairs
Assistant Professor
Department of Family Medicine
University of Medicine and Dentistry of New Jersey
School of Osteopathic Medicine
Stratford, NJ

Anthony S. Leazzo, D.O., FAAFP
Adjunct Clinical Faculty
Department of Family Medicine
Midwest University/Chicago College of Osteopathic Medicine
Downers Grove, IL
Team Physician, Joliet Buccaneers Football Club, Joliet, IL, and United States National Soccer Team, Chicago, IL

Robert Pedowitz, D.O.
Physician, Medical Director
Broadway Family Practice
Camden, New Jersey
Trenton Family Practice
Trenton, NJ

Craig Phelps, D.O., FAOASM
Provost
A.T. Still University of Health Sciences, Mesa
Team Physician, NBA Phoenix Suns, WNBA Phoenix Mercury, Ballet Arizona, Grand Canyon University, and Scottsdale Community College, Paradise Valley Community College and Gateway Community College

Richard G. Schuster, D.O.
Associate Professor
Department of Osteopathic Manual Medicine
Des Moines University College of Osteopathic Medicine
Des Moines, IA

Gail A. Shafer-Crane, Ph.D.
Assistant Professor
Department of Radiology
Michigan State University
East Lansing, MI

Alan R. Stockard, D.O., FAOASM
Past President, AOASM
Associate Professor
Department of Manipulative Medicine / Orthopedics
University of North Texas Health Science Center
Texas College of Osteopathic Medicine
Ft. Worth, TX

Jason M. Tarno, D.O., FAOASM
Crovetti Orthopaedics and Sports Medicine
Team Physician UNLV Athletics
Clinical Director University of Nevada School of Medicine Primary Care Sports Medicine Fellowship
Adjunct Faculty Touro University Nevada

Charles W. Webb, D.O.
Associate Professor Family Medicine & Orthopedics
Director Sports Medicine Program
Oregon Health & Science Center
Head Team Physician Portland State University and Lewis and Clark University, Portland, OR

J. Michael Wieting, D.O., MEd, FAOCPMR, FAAPMR
Professor
Physical Medicine and Rehabilitation and Osteopathic Manipulative Medicine
Director of Sports Medicine and Team Physician
Director of Program Development
Lincoln Memorial University-DeBusk College of Osteopathic Medicine
Harrogate, TN

Phillip Zinni III, D.O., FAOASM, ATC
Adjunct Faculty
Department of Family Practice
Touro University Nevada College of Osteopathic Medicine
Henderson, NV
CEO & Medical Director, Zinni Medical Institute
Las Vegas, NV
President, AOASM
National Medical Director, The Industrial Athlete
Rochester Hills, MI
Medical Director, Rock n' Roll Marathon – Las Vegas

1 The Cervical Spine Exam

Bernard King, D.O., FAOASM
Richard Schuster, D.O.

ANATOMY

The cervical spine, consisting of seven cervical vertebrae, furnishes stability and support for the head, permits motion of the head and neck, and provides protection and housing for the cervical spinal cord and nerve roots as well as the vertebral artery.

Beginning anteriorly, the horseshoe-shaped hyoid bone can be palpated in the crease of the neck superior to the thyroid cartilage at the level of the C3 vertebral body. Inferior to the hyoid bone in the midline of the neck is the thyroid cartilage. The superior notch can be palpated as well as the bulging central region, commonly referred to as the "Adam's apple." The thyroid cartilage lies at the level of the C4 and C5 vertebral bodies. It forms a complete ring, which is narrower anteriorly and considerably wider posteriorly. The cricothyroid membrane can be palpated between the thyroid and cricoids cartilages. Inferior to the cricoids cartilages is the first tracheal ring. The carotid tubercle lies about 2.5 cm lateral to the cricoids cartilage. This is the small anterior tubercle on the transverse process of the C6 vertebra and is covered by overlying muscles. The common carotid artery runs adjacent to the tubercle, and locating this tubercle is frequently used as a landmark for approaching the inferior cervical (stellate) sympathetic ganglion. The transverse process of the atlas (C1) can be palpated inferior to the ear between the angle of the mandible and the mastoid process of the temporal bone.

On the lateral aspect of the skull, about 4 cm superior to the midpoint of the zygomatic arch, is the pterion. This is an H-shaped formation of sutures that unites the frontal, parietal, sphenoid, and temporal bones. The pterion is important clinically because it overlies the anterior branches of the middle meningeal artery, and a blow to this vulnerable area may rupture the underlying vessels. Posterior landmarks begin with the occipital bone (occiput). On the occipital bone one can palpate the external occipital protuberance (inion) on the midline and the superior nuchal line extending laterally from the external occipital protuberance. At the lateral end of the superior nuchal line, the rounded mastoid process of the temporal bone can be palpated.

Beginning at the external occipital protuberance and proceeding inferiorly, the spinous processes of the cervical vertebrae can be palpated along the midline of the neck. The midline of the neck is indented due to the presence of the nuchal ligament lying immediately over the spinous processes and the laterally located paraspinal muscles and the overlying trapezius muscle. The first cervical spinous process that can be palpated is C2 and the rest can be palpated sequentially to C7.

All seven cervical vertebrae are easily identified by the presence of a transverse foramen in each transverse process. These foramina transmit the vertebral artery and accompanying sympathetic nerve plexus. Cervical vertebrae C3-C7 share common anatomic features. The uncus articulates with beveled reciprocal facets on the inferior surface of the vertebral body above to form the uncovertebral joints (of Luschka). The pedicles are short and, along with the lateral aspect of the body, serve as the origin for the broad transverse processes. The superior and inferior vertebral notches are shallow, thus creating a very narrow intervertebral foramen. The spinous processes of C2-C6 may or may not be bifid. The C7 spinous process is the longest and most prominent cervical spinous process.

The first two cervical vertebrae are adapted for movements of the head. The atlas, C1, is attached to, and "holds up," the skull. The axis, C2, provides the axis upon which the atlas and the attached skull can rotate. The atlas lacks a body and is composed of an anterior and posterior arch connected on each side to lateral masses. The lateral masses contain superior and inferior articular facets. The superior facets face superiorly and articulate with the occipital condyles of the occipital bones, while the inferior facets face inferiorly and articulate with the superior facets on the body of the axis. The internal surface of the anterior arch contains a small facet for the articulations with the dens of the axis. Projecting off of the anterior arch is an anterior tubercle, while projecting off of the posterior arch is the posterior tubercle, which replaces the spinous process. The transverse processes are prominent and contain the vertebral foramina. On the superior surface of the posterior arch is a groove for the vertebral artery as it crosses the arch to enter the vertebral canal. The axis consists of a body and a vertical dens projecting superiorly off of the body. The dens has anterior and posterior facets for articulation with the facet on the anterior arch of the atlas and the transverse ligament of the atlas. The axis has no superior articular processes, but does have superior articular facets on each side of the body. Its inferior articular processes, spinous process, and transverse processes resemble those of other cervical vertebrae.

In the cervical spine two types of joints, other than the uncovertebral joints described previously, unite cervical vertebrae C2-C7. These include facet joints (zygapophyseal joints) and intervertebral body joints (intervertebral discs). The facet joints are synovial joints between the articular processes of the adjacent vertebrae. A thin, loose articular capsule surrounds each joint. The facet joints permit gliding movements between the vertebrae, and the shape of the articular surfaces limits the range of motion possible. Branches arising from the posterior primary rami of the spinal nerves innervate these joints. The intervertebral discs are fibrocartilaginous joints, designed for weight bearing and strength, situated between the bodies of adjacent vertebrae. Each intervertebral disc consists of an outer anulus fibrosus, composed of concentric lamellae of fibrocartilage, which surrounds a gelatinous nucleus pulposus. The anuli insert into the rounded rims on the articular surfaces of adjacent vertebral bodies. Branches arising from the anterior primary rami of the spinal nerves innervate the intervertebral discs. The intervertebral discs are avascular structures, which receive their blood supply by diffusion from the vertebral bodies.

Ligaments reinforce and stabilize the facet joints and the intervertebral discs between the C2-C7 vertebrae. The anterior and posterior longitudinal ligaments resist anterior and posterior displacement of the vertebral bodies on one another. The anterior longitudinal ligament limits extension of the vertebral column. The posterior longitudinal ligament runs within the vertebral canal beginning at C2 and limits flexion of the vertebral column. The strong, highly elastic, flattened ligamentum flava attach to the laminae of adjacent vertebrae to preserve the normal curvature of the vertebral column after it has been flexed. Short interspinous ligaments join adjacent spinous processes. In the cervical spine, the supraspinous ligament is replaced by the ligamentum nuchae, which separates the muscles on each side of the posterior neck and provides attachment for them. On its deep service, it attaches to the spinous processes of the cervical vertebrae, while superiorly it attaches to the external occipital protuberance and median nuchal line. Its posterior margin spans the distance between the external occipital protuberance and the spinous process of C7. This ligament helps to support the weight of the head when it is flexed.

The atlanto-occipital facets are obliquely positioned and permit nodding of the head and some lateral bending with practically no rotation. The three atlantoaxial joints are specialized for head rotation. The median atlantoaxial joint is a pivot, with the atlas pivoting around the dens and carrying the head with it. Several strong ligaments provide the stability of the atlanto-occipital and atlantoaxial joints, most importantly the transverse ligament of the atlas, which converts the anterior arch of the atlas into a complete ring around the dens. The dens is connected to the occipital condyles of the occipital bone by the alar ligaments, which limit flexion and rotation. Extending superiorly and inferiorly from the transverse ligament of the atlas are superior and inferior crura, which together form a ligamentous complex referred to as the cruciform ligament.

The vertebral artery, which traverses the transverse foramina of the cervical vertebrae, typically arises from the subclavian artery at the base of the neck medial to the anterior scalene muscle. It runs superiorly and slightly posterior and usually enters the transverse foramen of the sixth cervical vertebra. Along with the artery are postganglionic sympathetic nerve fibers derived from the cervicothoracic or stellate ganglion and the vertebral vein. In the neck, small branches of the vertebral artery supply adjacent deep muscles of the neck and spinal branches enter the intervertebral foramina to supply the spinal cord and its coverings.

In the cervical spine two major functional groups of muscles are present: extensors and flexors. Each group is also capable of rotating and laterally bending the cervical spine. The extensor muscles are situated posterior to the laminae and transverse processes of the cervical vertebrae. These muscles also lie deep to the cervical portion of the thoracolumbar fascia, which separates them from more superficial muscles (trapezius and rhomboids) attaching the spine to the upper limb.

The extensor muscles can be divided into four groups: the splenius, erector spinae, transversospinalis, and suboccipital muscles. These muscles are arranged in three layers. The superficial layer contains the erector spinae and the splenius muscles. The intermediate layer contains the semispinalis and multifidus muscles of the transversospinalis group. The deep layer contains the interspinal, intertransverse, and rotator muscles of the transversospinalis group and the suboccipital muscles. The splenius muscles consist of the broad splenius capitis and the narrow splenius cervicis. The erector spinae muscles in the neck include the following from superficial to deep:

1. Iliocostalis cervicis
2. Longissimus capitis
3. Longissimus cervicis and capitis
4. Semispinalis cervicis and capitis

The multifidus muscles, lying deep to the semispinalis muscles, are thin in the cervical region. They arise from the articular processes of the lower four cervical vertebrae, run medially and superiorly and attach into the spinous processes of the axis and the upper two or three cervical vertebrae below the axis. The interspinous, intertransverse, and rotator muscles lie deep to the multifidus and are fairly well developed in the cervical region.

The suboccipital muscles connect the atlas and the axis to each other and to the skull and function in rotating and extending the head. This muscle group is composed of major and minor rectus muscles and superior and inferior oblique muscles. The rectus muscles produce extension of the atlanto-occipital joints, whereas the oblique muscles rotate the atlas and the skull on the axis. The major and minor oblique muscles and the major rectus muscle form the borders of the suboccipital triangle. This triangle contains the vertebral artery, suboccipital nerve, which supplies all of the suboccipital muscles and sensory greater occipital nerve.

The flexor muscles of the cervical spine are important in raising the head from a supine position. These prevertebral muscles in the cervical region are in close apposition to the vertebral column, directly flex the spine, and are represented by the longus colli and scalene muscles. The sternocleidomastoid muscle, attaching superiorly to the mastoid process of the skull and inferiorly to the manubrium of the sternum and the clavicle, is a more powerful flexor of the cervical spine than the prevertebral muscles because of its more anterior position. Not only does it draw the head forward but it also flexes the cervical spine. The sternocleidomastoid is also the most powerful rotator of the cervical spine but it works in combination with other muscles. The prevertebral muscles are innervated by the anterior primary rami of the cervical spinal nerves, while the sternocleidomastoid muscle is innervated by the accessory nerve (CN XI).

The spinal cord and its coverings (meninges) are located in the vertebral canal of the cervical spine. The cervical spine contains eight cervical spinal cord segments along with their anterior and posterior nerve roots. Cervical spinal nerves (eight pairs) are formed just outside the intervertebral formamina by the union of the anterior and posterior roots. In the cervical spine, the spinal nerves are formed above the vertebra they correspond to in number. Thus, the C1 spinal nerve is formed between the skull and the atlas, while the C8 spinal nerve is formed just outside the intervertebral foramen between the C7 and T1 vertebrae. After the spinal nerve is formed, it divides almost immediately into anterior and posterior primary rami. The posterior primary rami innervate segmentally skin and muscles of the back as well as the facet joints of the cervical spine. Communications between the anterior primary rami of the C1-C4 spinal nerves form the cervical plexus deep to the internal jugular vein and the sternocleidomastoid muscle in the neck. The phrenic nerve is the motor nerve to the diaphragm; it arises from the

C3-C5 roots and descends through the neck on the anterior surface of the anterior scalene muscle down to the diaphragm.

The brachial plexus is derived from the anterior primary rami of the C5-T1 spinal nerves and provides motor and sensory innervations to the upper limb. The plexus extends from the neck into the axilla and is composed of roots, trunk divisions, cords and branches. The roots and trunks with their branches lie in the posterior triangle of the neck, with the roots situated between the anterior and middle scalene muscles along with the subclavian artery. Branches in the neck include the dorsal scapular nerve (C5) to the rhomboid and levator scapulae muscles, the long thoracic nerve (C5-C7) to the serratus anterior muscle, and the suprascapular nerve (C5 and C6) running laterally across the posterior triangle of the neck to supply the supraspinatus and infraspinatus muscles and the shoulder joint.

There are several important soft tissue landmarks in the neck. The sternocleidomastoid muscle extends from the mastoid process of the skull to the manubrium of the sternum and clavicle, and divides the neck into anterior and posterior triangles. The muscle is palpable along its entire length. A lymph node chain is situated along the medical border of the sternocleidomastoid muscle. The trapezius muscle extends from the external occipital protuberance to the T12 vertebra and attaches laterally into the clavicle, the acromion, and the spine of the scapula. The muscle can be palpated along its superior border from its origin to its distal attachment. The trapezius and the sternocleidomastoid share a continuous attachment along the base of the skull to the mastoid process as well as a common nerve supply by way of the accessory nerve (CN XI). The superior border of the trapezius forms the posterior boundary of the posterior triangle of the neck. The thyroid gland lies in the anterior triangle of the neck at the level of the C5-T1 vertebrae. It consists of right and left lobes located anterolateral to the larynx and trachea on the midline of the neck at the level of the second to third tracheal rings. The esophagus, posterior to the trachea, begins at the inferior border of the thyroid cartilage and passes inferiorly through the superior thoracic aperture into the thorax. The carotid sheath is a fascial tube that extends from the base of the skull to the root of the neck deep to the sternocleidomastoid muscle in the anterior triangle of the neck. It contains the common and internal carotid arteries, internal jugular vein, and vagus nerve (CN X). At the level of the superior border of the thyroid cartilage, the common carotid artery divides into the internal and external carotid arteries. The root of the neck (supraclavicular fossa) is at the junction between the neck and the superior thoracic aperture. It is bounded anteriorly by the manubrium of the sternum, laterally by the first rib, and posteriorly by the body of the T1 vertebra. The sternocleidomastoid muscle, as it approaches its distal attachment, and covered by the platysma muscle, can be palpated.

HISTORY

As in all aspects of medicine, history taking is of great importance. With patients complaining of head, neck, trapezius or shoulder pain, full consideration should be given to the cervical spine as a source for their pain. Account should be taken of which sport or sports an athlete may be participating, as each sport often has its own injury pattern. A full description of the patient's symptoms should be sought, including onset, trauma, timing, evolution, distribution and nature of the symptoms.

Age is very important as some disorders have a predilection for certain age groups. For instance, radicular pain under the age of 35 is rarely caused by disc disease, except after trauma. In younger patients it is more commonly due to neurofibroma. In the elderly, radicular pain is more commonly related to compression by facet or uncovertebral joint hypertrophy. Torticollis in an infant is most often congenital, while in a young child, most often from swollen lymph nodes secondary to infection. Whenever symptoms occur in a patient of the 'wrong' age group, further investigation is always warranted.

Pain is the most common presenting symptom. Exact localization and distribution of the pain may give information toward localization of the lesion. Pain may be acute, subacute, chronic or recurrent. Acute or subacute pain tends not to be as common, except in young people following trauma. Chronic problems tend to wax and wane for months or years without much tendency toward self-resolution. Most commonly, though, patients present with recurrent symptoms, suggesting attacks of short duration. In these cases precise description of the symptoms is sought. How long do attacks typically last? Do they occur in typical patterns? Do the symptoms completely resolve after each attack, or are there residual symptoms?

One particularly worrisome symptom should be mentioned. A patient complaining of electrical shock sensations down the spine or both arms (Lhermitte's sign) may be an indication of severe cervical spinal canal stenosis. Should this symptom be elicited, further investigation should be initiated for spinal stenosis or the other entities that are part of the differential diagnosis for Lhermitte's sign (such as multiple sclerosis, amyotrophic lateral sclerosis, Arnold-Chiari malformation, et al.).

Onset of symptoms should be sought. Where did it start? When did it start? How did it start? All of these are particularly important. In order to understand these questions, one must understand the nature of dural pain. The dura is innervated by the sinuvertebral nerve, but with much cross innervation from several levels. This results in multisegmental pain referral pattern. Very often, pain of cervical origin is not felt in the neck, except initially, and therefore easily overlooked as a source for the patient's complaints. The classic example of this is mid-thoracic, interscapular pain, which is most often caused by a lower cervical disc compressing the dura. Pain in the neck often occurs initially, and then resolves to be followed by interscapular pain. Very often the patient has forgotten the initial neck pain unless such information is specifically asked about.

The next question to ask is "How have the symptoms changed?" This relates directly to the above questions. A progression from initial neck pain, to interscapular pain, to radicular pain down the arm, might describe a central disc herniation pressing on the dura, and then pressing against the dural sleeve of the exiting nerve root. Very often discogenic pain in the cervical spine is self-limited but recurrent. Pain that is constant, particularly lasting more than six months, would suggest another cause, such as synovial cyst or degenerative change, or a progressive cause such as metastasis.

Because most discogenic lesions are episodic, it is very helpful to know how the symptoms have changed, how the patient has responded to previous treatments, and how long they have lasted. Instability is a common factor in discogenic lesions. This results in pain that often changes from one side to another between episodes, but responds to the same treatment as previously. Often there is consistency to the duration of attacks as well. It is also common that between attacks there is complete resolution of pain. Lack of complete resolution requires a search for why treatment has failed, be it a failure of diagnosis or a failure of treatment.

Ascertainment of the details of current symptoms is the next step. Localization of the current symptoms is very important, but may vary from headache, to facial, neck, scapular, pectoral or arm pain. Headache or facial pain of cervical origin would suggest an upper cervical lesion between atlanto-occipital joint or the atlanto-axial joint. Pain to the vertex would suggest C1, while pain to the frontal region would suggest C2. Pain in the face would suggest a more local lesion (such as sinusitis, dental lesions, temporo-mandibular joint dysfunction, neoplasm, abscess, etc.), but can be referred from the neck, typically from C2, though also could be from a multisegmental origin. Pain in the scapular region is typically from a lower cervical origin. Rarely pectoral pain can be referred from the cervical spine in a multisegmental manner. Neck and arm pain are fairly straightforward.

Paresthesia is a common symptom. As a general rule, it should be considered much the same as pain when trying to determine a level of origination.

Vertigo can be associated with cervical spine disease. It is important to consider vertebral artery insufficiency when considering vertigo of cervical origin, but structural disease can often be involved. Presumably this relates to proprioceptive feedback from the muscles and ligaments, or to direct influence on the cervical sympathetic ganglia. Recently consideration of vagal influences has also been given attention.

PHYSICAL EXAM

Inspection

Inspection of the cervical spine should reveal sufficient cervical lordosis, or a backward curve (Figure 1.1). Loss of this curve may be a clue to the source of pain, such as degenerative disc disease or spondylosis. Poor posture, particularly in more mature patients with early spinal osteoarthritis or disc degeneration, leads to increased "humping" at the C6-T2 region. The head should sit between the shoulders, not in front of them. Note any abnormal rotation or side bending. When inspecting the patient from the front, the nose should be in line with the sternum. From the side, the earlobe should be in line with the acromion process. The muscle bulk of the trapezius, deltoid, and sternocleidomastoid muscles should be symmetrical; however, often the patient's dominant shoulder will lie lower than the non-dominant shoulder.

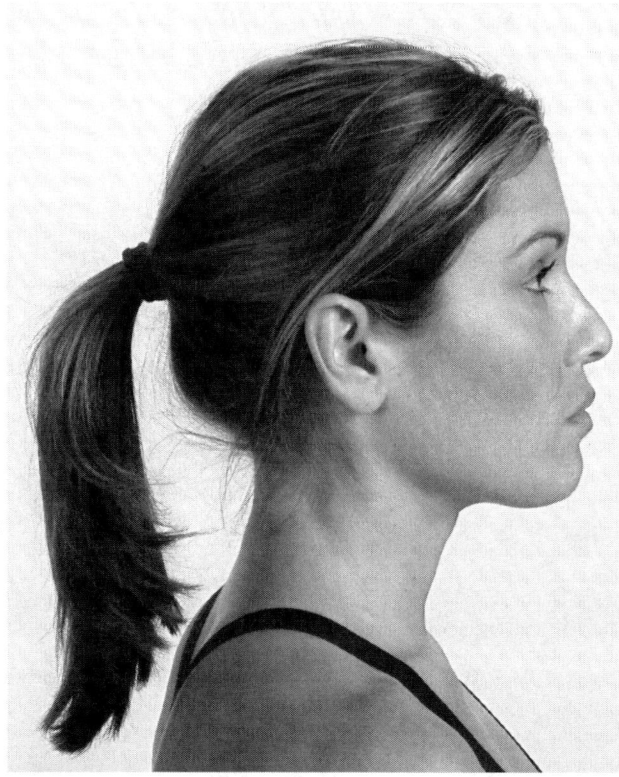

Figure 1.1. Lateral view of the cervical spine.

Palpation

Starting at the anterior cervical region superiorly, palpate the hyoid bone, thyroid cartilage (Figure 1.2), and first cricoids cartilage ring. The thyroid gland is just inferior and lateral to the thyroid cartilage, while the sternocleidomastoid lays just one fingerbreadth laterally from the thyroid gland. Palpate these structures, noting pain or deformity.

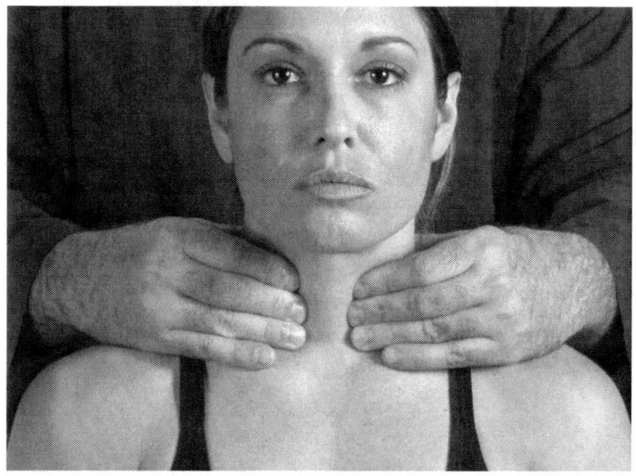

Figure 1.2. Palpation of the thyroid gland

At the base of the neck anteriorly, palpate the sternoclavicular (SC) joints and the length of the clavicles bilaterally, noting position, joint play, and motion. The position of the SC joints can be gauged by resting the index finger on the anterior-superior surfaces and comparing the finger positions. Passively elevate, rotate, and extend the patient's arm while monitoring the SC joint to further evaluate joint motion (Figure 1.3). The sternocleidomastoid inserts here as well, so palpate its enthesis for pain or disruption.

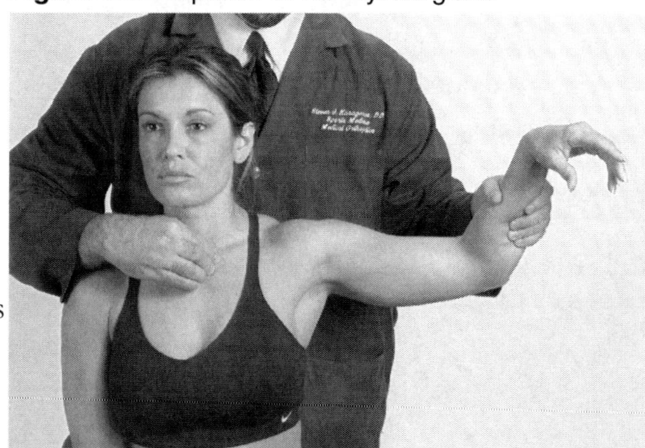

Figure 1.3. Palpation of the sternoclavicular joint while performing range of motion of the ipsilateral arm.

The cervical spine examination can be done with the patient supine to allow the neck muscles to relax, although the examination can also be done with the patient seated. The examiner should palpate the suboccipital fossae and note tenderness and somatic dysfunction. This is easier in the supine position. Traveling superolaterally from the fossae are the greater occipital nerves, which may be tender in patients with chronic headaches and in those with atlantoaxial and occipitoatlantal dyfunctions.

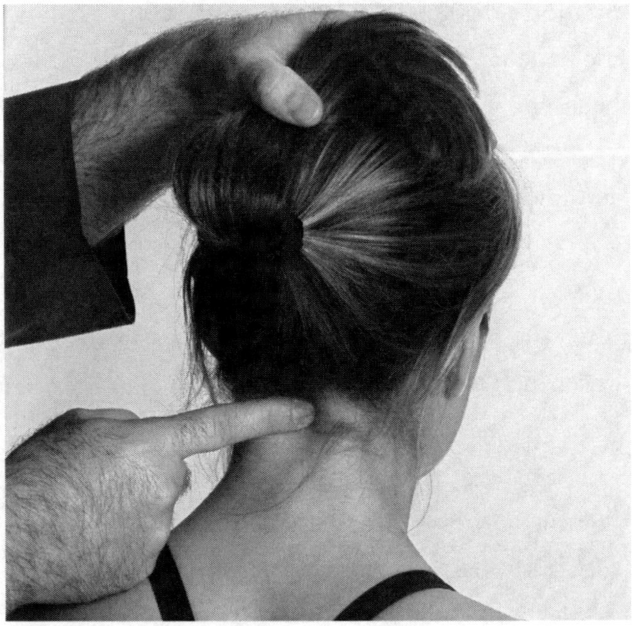

Figure 1.4. Palpation of the spinous process of C2 just inferior to the occiput.

The first palpable vertebral structure below the occiput is the spinous process of C2. Palpate along the spinous processes of C2 through C7, noting pain, swelling, stepoffs, and any differences in interspinous distance (Figure 1.4). Note the superior nuchal ligament and the interspinous ligaments during palpation, especially in injuries involving sudden hyperflexion of the neck. Palpate with the neck flexed as well.

The spinous processes of C6 and C7 should be more prominent than those of C3-C5, but the C6 prominence disappears when the neck is in extension. Any cervical spine with spinous processes that show either a stepoff or a significant difference in interspinous distance needs radiographs taken to rule out instability or fracture. The transverse process of C1 can be palpated inferior and anterior to the mastoid process.

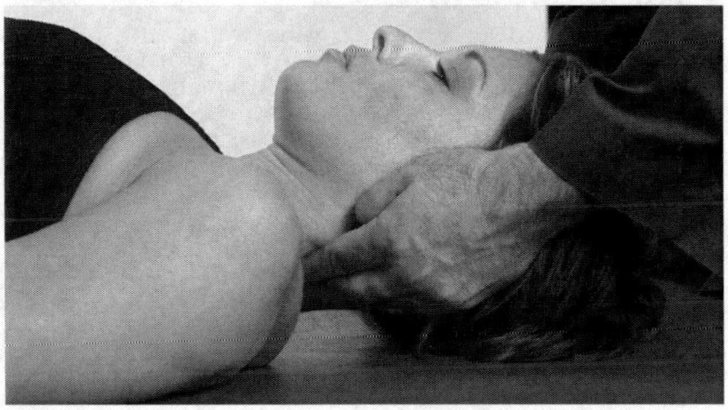

Figure 1.5. Palpation of the lateral cervical pillars.

Move laterally and palpate along the facet joints, noting any prominent pillars or tender points (Figure 1.5). Note whether one facet is more prominent than the one on the contralateral side, for this can help identify a somatic dysfunction. Finally, continue to move laterally and palpate the musculature in the posterior neck.

NOTE: In acute injuries or if the patient is unconscious, Palpation should always precede Range of Motion.

Range of Motion

Active Range of Motion

The examiner asks the patient to perform four motions:

1. Bend the head backward.
2. Bring the chin to the chest.
3. Look over the left and right shoulders.
4. Bring each ear to each shoulder (without cervical rotation).

Normal range of motion for the cervical spine is: flexion 60-90°; extension 70-90°; side bending 20-45°; rotation 70-90°. Cervical flexion primarily occurs at the occipitoatlantal joint and centers on the C5 and C6 vertebrae, while cervical extension centers around the C6 and C7 vertebrae. Rotation occurs primarily at the atlantoaxial joint. Side bending occurs primarily at the occipitoatlantal and atlantoaxial joints. Vertebrae C3 through C7 move in flexion and extension as one continuous group. While the patient is flexing, pay close attention to the spinous processes and note if any vertebral body is more prominent than the others. As each motion is carried out, information concerning reproduction of symptoms is sought.

Passive Range of Motion

Passive range of motion (PROM) should be evaluated and compared with active range of motion. This is best tested in the seated position. Although all motions can be assessed, passive flexion and side bending often add little to the diagnosis, unless active or passive flexion is the most painful motion. In this case, concern for nuchal rigidity (due to meningeal inflammation) or a possible dens fracture exists. All effort should be made to rule out these particularly worrisome findings. Passive extension and rotation should always be conducted, however, with notation of pain reproduction, amplitude of motion and end-feel. Typical end-feel is elastic, while abnormal end-feel might be hard or abrupt (indicating bony restriction such as osteoarthritis), empty (patient asks the examiner to stop due to pain, but the examiner feels that more motion is possible. Further forcing could lead to voluntary muscle contraction), crisp (involuntary muscle guarding at a local level, usually associated with disc protrusion), or muscle spasm (generalized involuntary spasm is never normal and warrants further investigation for a severe disorder).

Resisted Range of Motion/Strength Assessment

Resisted movements are typically as an isometric contraction. Rotation should always be tested at the least, though all motions may be tested, because it also gives information on motor conduction of the C1 nerve root (like scapular elevation, the major innervation is from the spinal accessory nerve, but contributions from C1 exist. This should never demonstrate painless weakness.). Movement may be painful, weak, or both. True muscle or tendon lesions of the cervical spine are extremely uncommon. In some acute situations, the patient has so much pain that any motion exacerbates the pain, thus obscuring the underlying problem.

Intersegmental Motion Testing

Occipitoatlantal Motion: The patient lies supine with the examiner sitting at the head of the table. The examiner's hands hold the patient's head while the index and middle fingers are placed on the suboccipital space. Note any motion restriction or palpable dysfunction in the occipital articulation. The examiner introduces lateral translation to the left and right, noting ease of motion (Figure 1.6). Greater ease of translation to the left is a diagnosis of side bent left, rotated right. Testing is repeated in flexion and extension of the head.

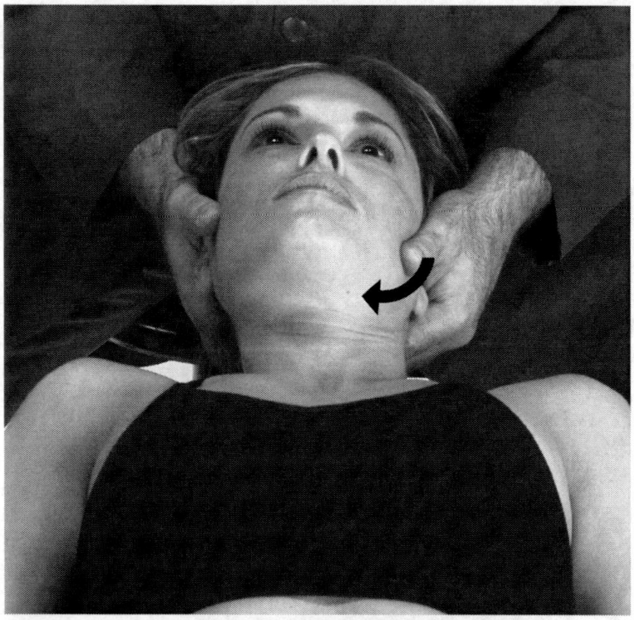

Figure 1.6. Occipitoatlantal motion.

Atlantoaxial Motion: With the patient supine, the examiner fully flexes the head while monitoring the lateral masses of the atlas with the index finger pads (flexion locks out the C2-C7 vertebrae). The head is rotated left and right, while the examiner notes any restriction or pain (Figure 1.7). If the head rotates farther to the left than the right, the diagnosis is AA rotated left.

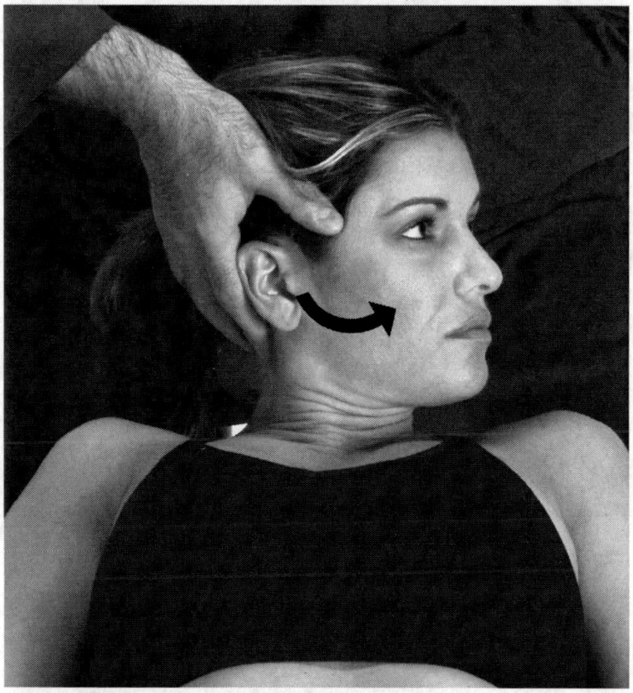

Figure 1.7. Atlantoaxial motion.

C2 through C7 Vertebrae: Intersegmental motion is more difficult to assess in the C2-C7 vertebrae, and the examiner will have more success palpating for joint play and tissue spring in each level. The examiner places the pads of the index fingers along the lateral side of the posterior pillars of the specific segment, while the rest of the hand supports the patient's head (Figure 1.8). The fingers introduce side bending into that segment, translating it left and right. Note spring, tenderness, and amount of play. Determine if a segment is restricted in the side-bending component.

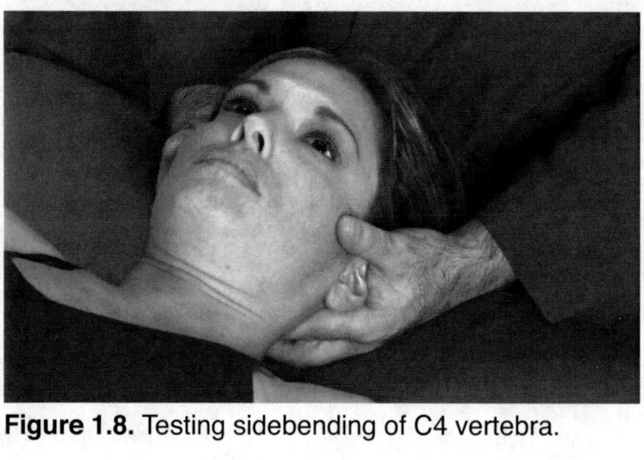

Figure 1.8. Testing sidebending of C4 vertebra.

Then palpate the posterior aspect of the facets introducing anterior translation to help identify a segmental extension restriction. Remember that C2-C7 vertebrae follow Type II (non-neutral) mechanics in obtaining a segmental diagnosis.

Neurovascular Examination

Neurological Examination: Deep tendon reflexes, muscle strength, and sensation of the upper extremities should be evaluated routinely. Deep tendon reflexes of the lower extremities should also be tested routinely as the presence of lower extremity hyperreflexia suggests an upper motor neuron lesion. Plantar response and clonus may need to be checked in selected cases. Other neurological tests should be done as clinically indicated.

Deep tendon reflexes are checked at the brachioradialis (C5), biceps (C5-6), and triceps (C7).

Muscle strength is assessed at the following levels: scapular elevation (C2-4), shoulder abduction (C5), elbow flexion (C5-6), wrist extension (C6), wrist flexion (C7), elbow extension (C7), thumb extension (C8), finger flexion (C8), and finger abduction (T1).

Sensation is assessed typically by pinprick over the different dermatomes, comparing one arm to the other. Because there is much overlap between the dermatomes, and much variation from person to person, comparison should be made from the unaffected side to the affected side, in order to achieve reliable information.

Carotid Pulse: Palpate just medial to the mid-portion of the sternocleidomastoid muscle belly anteriorly. Note strength and rate of pulsation.

Jugulovenous Distention: Lay the patient back at 30 degrees and 60 degrees to observe jugular distention and pulsation. Pulses should be seen upon contraction of the heart, but the jugular veins should not be distended in either position after the upstroke. Evidence of distention should be investigated for causes such as fluid overload or heart failure.

Lymph Nodes: Palpate the nodes in the head and neck region, noting pain, enlargement, or erythema. The following regions should be evaluated for lymphadenopathy:

- Occipital nodes (skull base)
- Postauricular nodes superficial over the mastoid processes
- Preauricular nodes in front of the ear
- Parotid and retropharyngeal (tonsillar) nodes at the angle of the mandible
- Submaxillary nodes halfway between the angle and tip of the mandible
- Submental nodes behind the tip of the mandible
- Superficial cervical nodes near the sternocleidomastoid (SCM) muscle
- Posterior cervical nodes along the anterior border of the trapezius muscle
- Deep to the SCM
- Supraclavicular nodes in the region marked by the SCM and clavicle

PROVOCATIVE TESTS

Lhermitte's Sign. While simply sitting on the exam table and attempting to actively hold their head upright, the patient complains of electrical shock sensations down the spine or down both arms.

Indicates: Possible spinal stenosis (R/O MS, ALS, Arnold-Chiari malformation, etc.).

Spurling's Test. This is one of the most commonly performed neck tests. It is used to test for foraminal compression on a nerve root. The examiner extends the patient's neck, rotates the head to one side, and applies axial compression downward on the head (Figure 1.9).

Positive Test: Pain radiating down the arm to which the head is rotated.

Indicates: Cervical radiculopathy.

NOTE:. The provocative tests of Adson and Wright and the costoclavicular test are commonly done next, each indicating a different level of impingement on the subclavian artery.

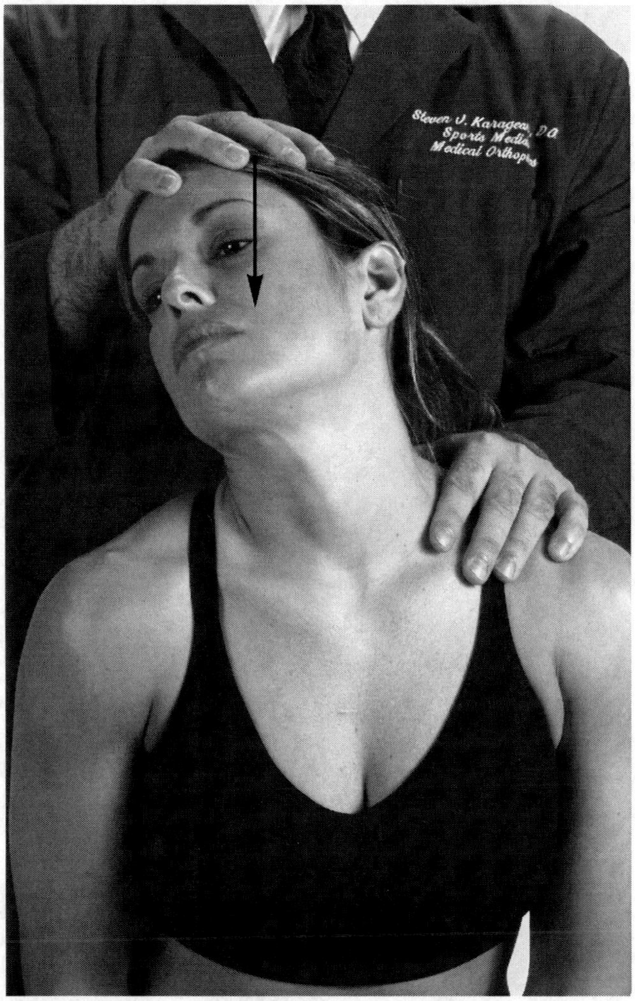

Figure 1.9. Spurling's Test.

Adson's Test. The examiner palpates the patient's radial pulse while lifting the arm into 90° abduction, and approximately 90° external rotation. The patient is asked to inhale and turn the head toward the affected side (Figure 1.10).

Positive Test: Reproduction of the patient's symptoms and/or a loss or marked diminution of the pulse.

Indicates: Impingement of the subclavian artery in the scalene triangle.

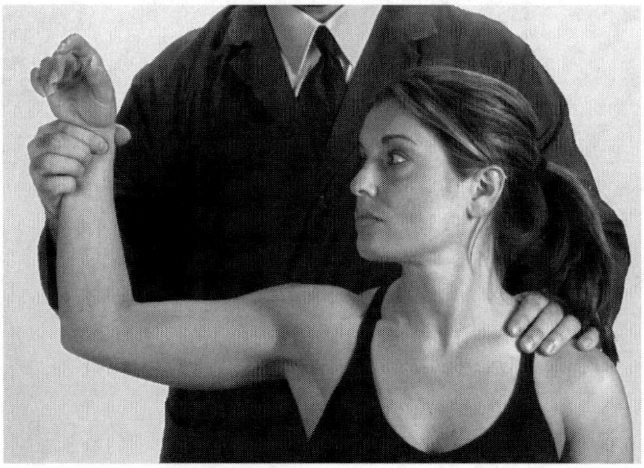
Figure 1.10. Adson's Test.

Wright's Test (also known as the Hyperabduction Test). The examiner palpates the patient's radial pulses bilaterally, while lifting the arms into full (180°) abduction.

Positive Test: Reproduction of the patient's symptoms and/or a loss or marked diminution of the pulse.

Indicates: Impingement of the subclavian artery by the pectoralis minor muscle.

Costoclavicular Test. The examiner palpates the patient's radial pulses bilaterally while asking the patient to extend and hang his arms off the back of the table.

Positive Test: Reproduction of the patient's symptoms and/or a loss or marked diminution of the pulse.

Indicates: Impingement of the subclavian artery beneath the clavicle.

Dural Tension Signs. There are no good dural tension signs for the cervical spine as there are for the lumbar spine (such as straight leg raising). Although scapular movements are typically part of the shoulder girdle examination, they can also be dural tension signs, particularly scapular retraction. The resisted motion of scapular elevation gives information on motor conduction of the C2-4 nerve roots (see note above on resisted cervical rotation). This motion should also never demonstrate weakness.

COMMON CONDITIONS

- Soft Tissue Injuries/Conditions
  - Cervical strain, cervical sprain
  - Cervical somatic dysfunction
  - Headache
  - Stingers/Burners
- Hard Tissue Injuries/Conditions
  - Osteoarthritis
  - Degenerative disc disease

Soft Tissue Injuries/Conditions

Cervical strain, cervical sprain: This is the most common of all of the cervical injuries and clearly the most common that the examiner will encounter. These conditions result when the soft tissue activity threshold is surpassed. Usually self-limited, the standard anti-inflammatory, ice, relative rest, gradual return to motion, graded physical therapy, and manipulative therapy will aid in the rehabilitation.

Headache: Otherwise known as cephalgia, this is a common condition that is essentially "head pain." Direct or indirect trauma can cause the scalp to have pain. Treatment is directed at relieving the soft tissue pain.

Stinger/Burners: These conditions result from either ipsilateral compressive or contra-lateral traction phenomena to the cervical plexus. The resultant pain travels down the corresponding nerve root producing pain and dysfunction accordingly. Treatment is usually a self-limiting, conservative protocol. Physical therapy can be applied to more resistant cases.

Hard Tissue Injuries/Conditions

Osteoarthritis: The common condition whereby the multiple joints and vertebral bony components develop the classic changes associated with osteoarthritis. Treatment is conservative and almost invariably involves anti-inflammatory medication and heat.

Degenerative disc disease: This is the common condition that results from the wear and tear phenomena that occur across the disc-vertebrae interface. DDD is usually associated with aging and the inherent loss of water content within the disc itself. Treatment is also directed at pain relief, anti-inflammatories, improved range of motion, and improved strength.

CONDITIONS THAT SHOULD NOT BE MISSED DUE TO MORBIDITY OR MORTALITY

- Fracture
- A-O disruption
- Herniated Disc
- Transient Quadriplegia

Fracture

Trauma induced damage that results from the violation of the force-threshold of the bony architecture of the cervical spine components. These diagnoses cannot be missed and must be in the differential of any condition in which moderate forces are at play, when pain and dysfunction are disproportional to the physical findings, when there is a neurologic finding, when there is pinpoint tenderness, or when the clinical suspicion is high. Fracture types include an unstable fracture, vertebral body fracture, or a complex fracture. Fractures found in the cervical spine should be considered an emergency until proven otherwise and always warrant further consult.

A-O Disruption

This condition occurs when the atlanto-occipital ligament is ruptured either through trauma or a congenital anomaly. The absence of the integrity of the ligament yields an unstable cervical spine.

Herniated Disc

This condition is the result of long-standing wear and tear or from the acute violation of the annulus whereby the soft nucleus pulposis is extruded onto surrounding neurologic structures. This results in neurologic compromise to those structures, resulting in radiating pain to the upper extremity. Treatment can range anywhere from the above conservative protocol to more aggressive interventions such as surgery, nucleoplasty, epidural injections, or nerve blocks.

Transient Quadriplegia

This condition is relatively uncommon. It results from an impingement to the cervical cord, producing a temporary neurapraxia to the four extremities. While it by definition is self-limited, physical therapy to strengthen the supportive muscular structures can help in reducing the rate of recurrence.

REFERENCES

1. Karageanes SJ. *Principles of Manual Sports Medicine.* Philadelphia, PA: Lippincott Williams & Wilkins; 2005.

2 The Shoulder Exam

Douglas Dietzel, D.O.
Anthony Leazzo, D.O.
Alan Stockard, D.O., FAOASM

ANATOMY

The shoulder joint is a ball-in-socket joint, but not a typical example of such in that the ball is much larger than the socket. This results in an intrinsic instability and hence the joint relies on static and dynamic soft tissue stabilizers to remain centered.

The static stabilizers include the: glenohumeral joint capsule, which is made up of the superior, middle and inferior glenohumeral ligaments. The dynamic stabilizers consist of anteriorly, the deltoid and pectoralis major muscles; posteriorly the latissimus dorsi and teres major muscles; and muscles of the rotator cuff, the supraspinatus, infraspinatus, subscapularis, and the teres minor. The stabilizers function to compress the convexity of the humeral head into the concavity of the glenoid (similar to a golf ball on a tee) as the major muscles move the humerus.

The shoulder girdle is composed of three joints and two articulations[1], which work together to permit movement of the upper limb. These include the sternoclavicular, the acromioclavicular, the glenohumeral (shoulder) joints, and the scapulothoracic, and acromiohumeral articulation.

Several bony structures can be palpated as one examines the shoulder girdle. Beginning on the midline is the suprasternal notch situated along the superior margin of the manubrium of the sternum. Immediately lateral to the suprasternal notch is the sternoclavicular joint. The medial end of the clavicle participates in this joint and lies slightly superior to the manubrium. The sternoclavicular joint is divided into two compartments by an articular cartilage. The medial end of the clavicle articulates with the manubrium of the sternum and the first costal cartilage, reinforced by the anterior and posterior sternoclavicular ligaments. The sternoclavicular joint moves in anterior, posterior, superior, and inferior directions. Moving laterally from the sternoclavicular joint one can palpate the smooth superior surface of the clavicle, which is covered by the thin platysma muscle. The medial two thirds of the clavicle are convex, while the lateral one third is concave. At the deepest point of the concavity of the clavicle, inferior and deep to the anterior edge, the coracoid process of the scapula can be palpated. The coracoid process faces anterolaterally, lies deep to the pectoralis minor muscle, and may be felt by palpating into the deltopectoral triangle.

At the lateral end of the clavicle is the subcutaneous acromioclavicular joint. It is here where the clavicle, which has begun to flatten out, protrudes slightly above the acromion process of the scapula. The acromion is rectangular in shape, contributes to the contour of the shoulder, and can be palpated on its superior and anterior surfaces. The acromioclavicular joint is a synovial joint, surrounded by an articular capsule, where the lateral end of the clavicle articulates with the acromion of the scapula. The acromion rotates on the clavicle from scapulothoracic movements.

Posteriorly, the acromion tapers and continues as the spine of the scapula. The spine extends obliquely across the superior four fifths of the posterior surface of the scapula and ends as a flat triangle on the vertebral border of the scapula at the level of T3. The vertebral border, lying approximately 5 cm from the spinous process of the thoracic vertebrae, terminates superiorly at the superior angle, which is covered by the levator scapulae muscle. The vertebral border ends inferiorly at the subcutaneous inferior angle. The lateral border, which is covered by the latissimus dorsi, teres major, and teres minor muscles, runs obliquely towards the glenoid.

Laterally and inferiorly from the lateral lip of the acromion, the greater tubercle of the humerus can be felt. The bicipital groove of the humerus is situated anterior and medial to the greater tubercle. It is bordered laterally by the greater tubercle and medially by the lesser tubercle. It is best palpated with the arm laterally rotated. Within the bicipital groove is the tendon of the long head of the biceps muscle. Inferior to the acromion is the shoulder joint, which cannot be palpated. This is a very mobile joint where the head of the humerus fits into a very shallow glenoid cavity. As a result, the humerus is suspended from the scapula by muscles, ligaments, and a loose joint capsule with very little bony support.

The glenohumeral joint is a synovial joint where the head of the humerus articulates with the shallow glenoid cavity of the scapula, which is deepened by the fibrocartilaginous glenoid labrum. The loose joint capsule is attached medially to the margin of the glenoid cavity and laterally to the anatomic neck of the humerus. The synovial lining of the capsule forms a sheath for the tendon of the long head of the biceps muscle, which runs through the joint cavity.

The rotator cuff muscles attach the scapula to the humerus. The supraspinatus, infraspinatus, and teres minor are palpable at their attachments onto the greater tubercle of the humerus. The supraspinatus is an abductor of the humerus, while the infraspinatus and teres minor are lateral (external) rotators. With the arm hanging at the side, the supraspinatus lies directly over the head of the humerus deep to the acromion. The infraspinatus is posterior and inferior to the supraspinatus, and the teres minor is posterior and inferior to the infraspinatus. The fourth cuff muscle, the subscapularis, lies anterior to and on the undersurface of the scapula attaching to the lesser tubercle of the humerus, and acts as a medial (internal) rotator of the humerus.

The supraspinatus is innervated by the suprascapular nerve, the infraspinatus by the suprascapular nerve, the teres minor by the axillary nerve, and the subscapularis by the upper and lower subscapular nerve.

Bursae surround the shoulder lying between the tendons of the rotator cuff muscles and the shoulder joint capsule. They reduce friction on the tendons passing over bones and other areas of resistance. The subacromial bursa lies between the tendon of the supraspinatus muscle and the overlying acromion process of the scapula. Several portions of this bursa are palpable. A lateral extension of the subacromial bursa, the subdeltoid bursa, extends deep to the deltoid muscle, separating it from the rotator cuff below and allowing each to move more freely.

Several other muscles attach to the shoulder girdle and can be palpated. The sternocleidomastoid muscle arises from the manubrium of the sternum and the medial third of the clavicle, bisects the neck obliquely, and attaches superiorly to the mastoid process of the temporal bone. This muscle laterally flexes the neck and rotates the head to the opposite side and is innervated by the spinal accessory nerve.

The fan-shaped pectoralis major muscle forms the anterior wall of the axilla, arises from the medial two thirds of the clavicle and the anterior surfaces of the sternum, and inserts into the lateral lip of the bicipital groove of the humerus. It adducts and medially rotates the humerus, and draws the scapula anteriorly and inferiorly. The pectoralis major receives innervation from the lateral and medial pectoral nerves.

The biceps muscle, located in the anterior compartment of the arm, is composed of two heads, the long head and short head. The long head runs through the bicipital groove of the humerus and the shoulder joint cavity to attach to the supraglenoid tubercle of the scapula. The short head attaches to the coracoid process. Both heads attach distally to the radial tuberosity in the forearm. The biceps muscle supinates the forearm. It also flexes the supinated forearm. It receives its innervation from the musculocutaneous nerve.

The deltoid muscle contributes to the full contour of the shoulder and is divided into three parts. The anterior part of the muscle flexes and medially rotates the arm, the middle abducts the arm, and the posterior extends and laterally rotates the arm. The deltoid muscle is innervated by the axillary nerve.

The trapezius muscle is prominent in the cervical region. Its fibers attach onto the shoulder girdle at the lateral one third of the clavicle, the acromion, and the spine of the scapula. The main actions of this muscle are elevation-depression, retraction, and rotation of the scapula. The trapezius muscle is innervated by the spinal accessory nerve.

The axilla is at the junction of the arm and the thorax. The apex lies between the first rib, clavicle, and superior edge of the subscapularis muscle. Arteries, veins, lymphatics, and nerves pass through the apex connecting the arm and base of the neck. The pectoralis major muscle forms the anterior wall of the axilla; the posterior wall is formed chiefly by the latissimus dorsi muscle. The second through sixth ribs, and the overlying serratus anterior muscle define the medial wall. The lateral wall is the bicipital groove of the humerus containing the tendon of the long head of the biceps muscle. The brachial plexus arises from C5-T1 nerve roots and forms the origin of the major nerves to the upper limb. It runs in the axilla along with the axillary artery and its branches, the axillary vein and its tributaries, and axillary lymph nodes.

The rhomboid (major and minor) muscles are postural muscles. These muscles retract the scapula and rotate it to depress the glenoid cavity as well as fixing the scapula to the thoracic wall. They are innervated by the dorsal scapular nerve (C4, C5).

The latissimus dorsi muscle forms the posterior wall of the axilla. The latissimus dorsi extends, adducts, and medially rotates the humerus and is innervated by the thoracodorsal nerve (C6, C7, and C8).

The serratus anterior muscle can be palpated along the medial wall of the axilla. It originates from the external surfaces of the lateral aspects of the first to eighth ribs and attaches along the length of the anterior surface of the vertebral border of the scapula. The serratus anterior muscle is important in holding the scapula against the thoracic wall as well as in helping in scapular protraction and rotation. This muscle is innervated by the long thoracic nerve.

Table 2.1. Muscles of the Shoulder

Muscle	Origin	Insertion	Innervation
Platysma	Fascia covering superior aspect of pectoralis major and deltoid muscles	Symphysis menti, Mandible, Subcuticular facial fascia	Cervical branch of the facial nerve.
Supraspinatus	Scapula	Greater tubercle of the humerus	Suprascapular nerve
Infraspinatus	Scapula	Greater tubercle of the humerus	Suprascapular nerve
Teres Minor	Scapula	Greater tubercle of the humerus	Axillary nerve
Subscapularis	Scapula	Lesser tubercle of the humerus	Upper and lower subscapular nerve
Sternocleidomastoid	Manubrium, Medial 1/3 of clavicle	Mastoid	Spinal accessory nerve
Pectoralis major	Medial 2/3 of clavicle, Anterior sternum	Lateral lip of bicipital groove	Medial and lateral pectoral nerves
Biceps-Long head	Supraglenoid tubercle	Radial tuberosity	Musculocutaneous nerve
Biceps-Short head	Coracoid process	Radial tuberosity	Musculocutaneous nerve
Deltoid	Lateral clavicle, Lateral acromion, Posterior spine of scapula	Deltoid tuberosity	Axillary nerve
Rhomboid major	Spinous process of T2-T5, Supraspinatus ligament	Medial border of scapula	Doral scapular nerve
Rhomboid minor	Ligamentum nuchae, Spinous process of C7	Medical border of scapula	Doral scapular nerve
Latissimus dorsi	Spinous process of T6-T12, Posterior ilium, Supraspinous ligament, Thoracolumbar fascia	Inferior portion of the intertubercular groove	Thoracodorsal nerve
Serratus anterior	External and lateral surface of the 8th rib	Length of the anterior surface of the medial scapula	Long thoracic nerve
Trapezius	External occipital protuberance, Medial 1/3 superior nuchal line, Ligamentum nuchae, Spinous process of C7, Spinous process of T1-T12	Lateral 1/3 of the clavicle, Acromion, Spine of the scapula	Spinal accessory nerve

PHYSICAL EXAMINATION

The examination always begins with a thorough history. This leads to a specific physical examination with provocative tests/maneuvers for evaluation of the suspected condition.

Shoulder pain can be primary or referred from the cervical or thoracic areas, and occasionally from the heart as viscerosomatic pain, as in the case of angina or myocardial infarction.

Therefore, the history should include questions about the onset of the pain. Was it acute or gradual? If the pain was acute, was there an associated pop? If so, inquire about hearing or feeling more than one pop (a popping-out and popping-back-in sensation) that would suggest subluxation or dislocation. Ask about associated numbness, tingling, or burning pain distally along the upper extremity. Inquire about falls or trauma onto the tip of the shoulder or onto a flexed elbow or an outstretched arm.

If the patient is involved in a throwing or racquet sport, the phase of the activity when the pain occurs, such as the cocking phase, acceleration phase, release phase, or follow-through becomes paramount in determining the nature of the injury. Ask about any crepitance or a feeling of looseness since the injury. The clinician should access the quality of pain: sharp or dull, radiating or localized, intermittent or constant, worse with certain ranges of motion or activities such as throwing or raising the arms, i.e., what makes the pain worse or better.

When starting the physical examination of the shoulder, always examine the cervical spine as well. Even if the history is classic for an isolated shoulder injury, cervical pathology may be implicated, especially if the shoulder is targeted for treatment and the neck is not.

Observation

Whenever possible, observe the patient in a situation where he or she is unaware that they are being watched. Otherwise, observe the patient entering the examination room. Observe the patient's movement of the arms as he or she walks, sits on the examination table, etc. Many times, the examiner's first encounter with the patient is when he or she is seated on the examination table. Watch how the patient extends his or her hand to give a handshake and how he/she removes outer garments.

Expose both shoulders. The examiner should observe the anterior view with close attention to the acromion heights, the sternoclavicular and acromioclavicular joints, and the deltoid, pectoral, and anterior trapezius muscles (Figure 2.1). The bicipital groove and biceps muscle belly should be observed for deformity and swelling. In a lateral view, look for an increase in thoracic kyphosis, uneven scapulae, and/or winging of the scapulae. Also check proper alignment of the ear with the acromion process to rule out a cervical postural issue.

Posteriorly, look for a low shoulder or uneven scapulae by checking the acromion processes and the inferior angles of the scapulae. Note any hypertrophy or atrophy of the posterior shoulder girdle musculature. It is not uncommon to find hypertrophy in the dominant extremity, especially in throwing or racquet sport athletes. Examine the trapezius, levator scapulae, and rhomboid muscle groups for symmetry with the scapula. Note any scapular winging.

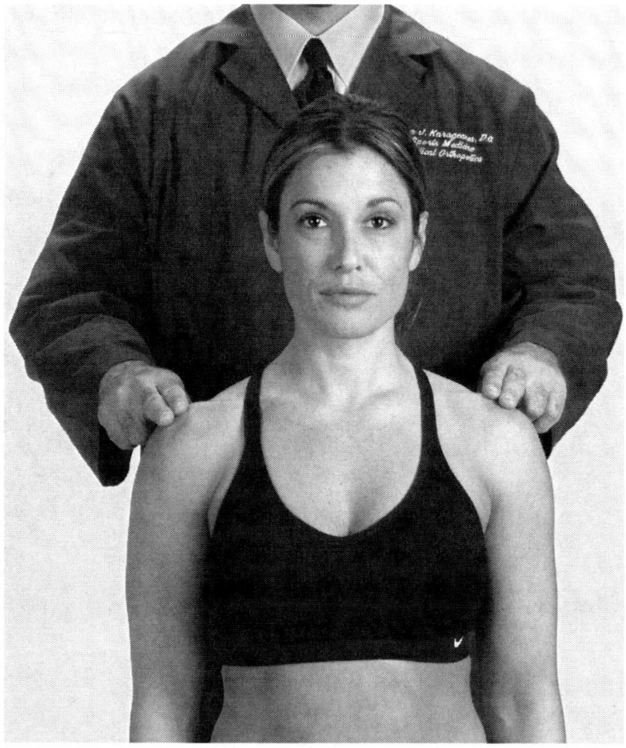

Figure 2.1. Evaluation of shoulder heights.

On inspection, also note indentations, nodules, or skin changes such as discoloration, hematomas, abrasions, and erythema. Scars, either postsurgical or otherwise, should be noted. Look for deformities from such conditions as glenohumeral dislocation (subacromial indentation), clavicular fractures, and acromioclavicular sprains. The scapulothoracic relationship should be noted. The scapula may be either retracted, protracted, or exhibit uneven heights.

Palpation

Begin by systematically palpating the bony prominences, and the muscles and tendons of the shoulder and the scapulothoracic region. Palpation should be aimed at eliciting tenderness, as well as TART changes. Be sure to palpate deeply enough to elicit pain. Test bilaterally in order to have a comparison.

An indentation posterior to the glenohumeral joint may suggest an anterior glenohumeral joint dislocation. The greater tuberosity of the humerus should be easily palpated (Figure 2.2). Significant palpable tenderness on bony prominences would cause the clinician to order radiographic studies to rule out fracture.

Palpation of the muscles should target the pectoralis, biceps brachii, deltoid (anterior, mid, and posterior portions), supraspinatus, the infraspinatus, teres minor, trapezius, and rhomboids posteriorly, and the latissimus dorsi, which comprises the posterior axilla. The sternocleidomastoid muscle should also be evaluated, as it is the most superior muscle involved in shoulder motion.

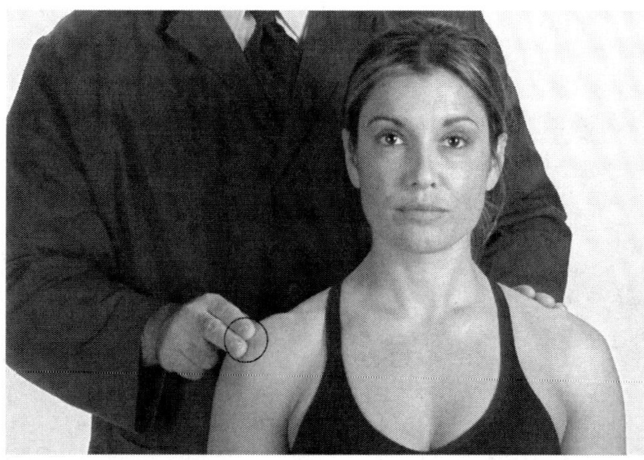

Figure 2.2. Palpation of greater tuberosity of humerus.

Palpate the tendons of the shoulder, specifically, the supraspinatus and the bicipital tendons. The subacromial bursa can also be palpated in most patients. This can be done seated or standing. To palpate the supraspinatus tendon at the greater tubercle, internally rotate the arm with the humerus at the side and elbow flex at 90 degrees (Figure 2.3). The biceps tendon can be palpated between the greater and lesser tubercles of the humerus (Figure 2.4). External rotation of the humerus allows the subscapularis to be palpated at the lesser tubercle (Figure 2.5). Palpate all muscle bellies and attachments at the scapula, acromion, crest of the scapula, and thoracic wall.

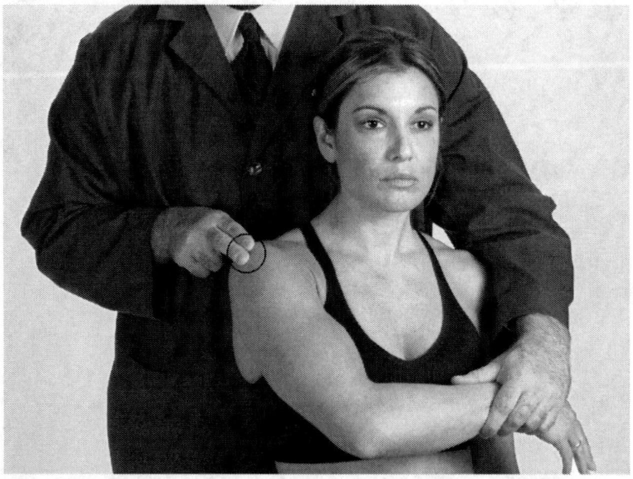

Figure 2.3. Palpation of Supraspinatus.

Range of Motion

When possible, observe ROM bilaterally to detect subtle differences. The shoulder should be actively and passively assessed in the following ranges:

NOTE: Several texts list various degrees of normal ROM, but these ranges are generally accepted.

- Abduction—arms at the side, elevate directly upward, and above the head. 0-180 degrees.
- Adduction—arm at 90-degree elevation, brought across the chest. 0-130 degrees.
- Flexion—arms at side, lifted in front of the patient over the head. 0-180 degrees.
- Extension—arms at side, brought straight back behind the patient. 0-60 degrees.
- Internal rotation posteriorly—arm at side, elbow flexed at 90 degrees, rotate arm in and bring behind back. 0-60-70 degrees.
- External rotation—arm at side, elbow flexed 90 degrees, rotate arms outward. 0-90 degrees.
- Scapular retraction—squeeze scapula together (bilaterally equal).
- Scapular protraction—reach forward

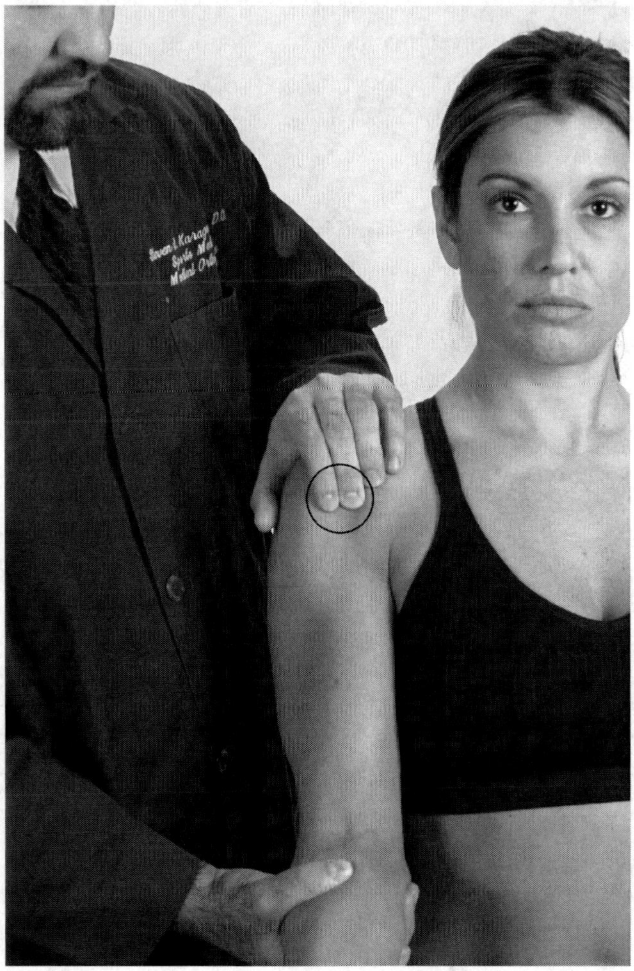

Figure 2.4. Palpation of biceps tendon.

- with both arms while observing scapular motion
- Scapular elevation—shoulder shrug (bilaterally equal).
- Rotation in abduction—Arm abducted to 90 degrees, elbow flexed to 90 degrees, rotate forearm into external rotation (90 degrees) and internal rotation (90 degrees).

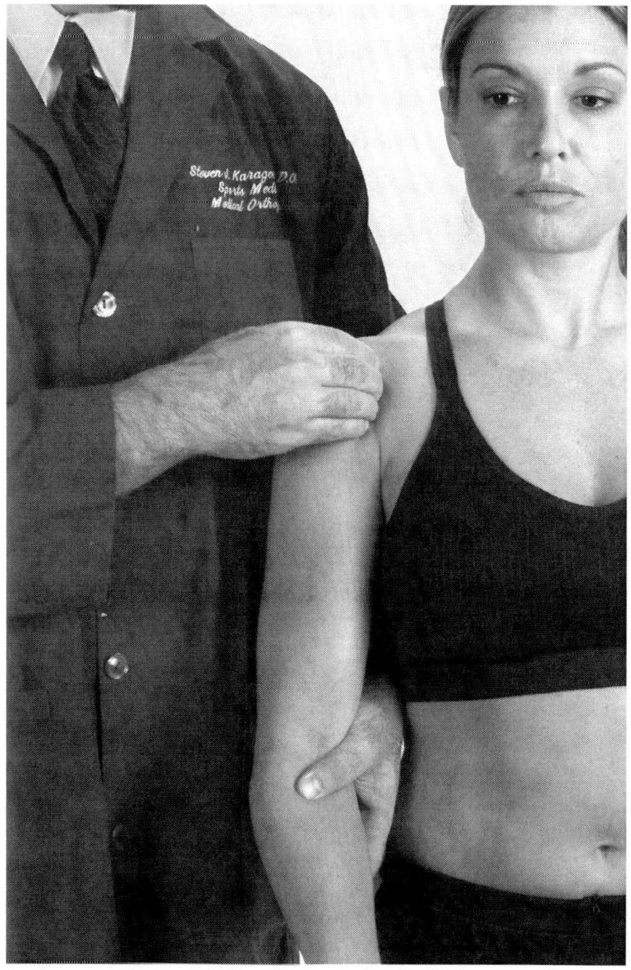

Figure 2.5. Palpation of subscapularis.

Note the range of motion and end-feel, as well as symptoms of instability, apprehension, and pain. If the active range of motion is limited, the examiner should assess the passive range of motion more carefully. Often the limiting factors of active range of motion are partial injuries that the examiner does not want to worsen by being too aggressive with his/her active examination. For instance, "sticking points" in a passive range of motion may identify a mechanical barrier such as a labral tear, rotator cuff tear, or adhesion formation. Pain can limit a patient's active range of motion, but if there is no mechanical barrier, then the examiner should be able to passively move the shoulder past that end point. Make sure the patient is relaxed during passive range of motion. Note any popping, clicking, or crepitus perceived by the patient or noted by the examiner.

There is quite a range of normal variance in the population. Some patients may have flexibility that would suggest possible capsular laxity but is normal for that particular patient. As with most "loose-jointed" individuals, this could predispose the patient to injury. Always compare both shoulders to distinguish general laxity from unilateral specific instability.

Look for glenohumeral motion isolated from scapulothoracic motion. Test the first 30 to 40 degrees of movement by having the patient raise both arms from his or her side overhead with straight elbows. Normally, the scapula will not start to rotate until the arm is abducted beyond 30 degrees. If abduction occurs with the shoulders shrugging, the patient is using scapulothoracic motion to compensate for glenohumeral restriction. If shrugging is not noted, glenohumeral motion is likely independent and normal (Figure 2.6).

Glenohumeral restriction is best seen in cases of adhesive capsulitis. Normally, the scapula rotates 1 degree for every 2 degrees of abduction at the glenohumeral joint. In a frozen shoulder, glenohumeral motion is markedly reduced, so abduction comes almost exclusively from scapular motion.

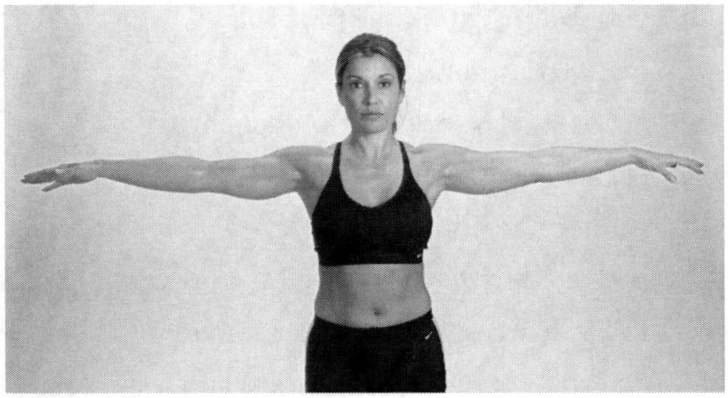

Figure 2.6. Normal scapulothoracic motion to 90 degrees of vertical abduction.

Apley's Scratch Test: There are two Apley's scratch maneuvers, the upper and the lower. These maneuvers help to determine range of motion. It should be noted that most patients have inequality with this maneuver, in that most patients normally have one shoulder that is somewhat tighter than the other. The lower test grossly checks internal rotation, adduction, and extension. The upper test checks for external rotation, abduction, and flexion.

Lower test: The patient puts the arm behind his or her back with the palm facing outward and the thumb pointed cephalad. The patient should then elevate the thumb as high as possible on the back while the examiner notes the level on the spine at which the thumb can reach (Figure 2.7). At this point, the Liftoff Test can be done if desired (Figure 2.8).

Upper test: The patient abducts the arm, placing the palm of the hand behind the neck with palm facing toward his or her body. The patient should then attempt to scratch the lowest possible vertebrae with the index finger (Figure 2.9).

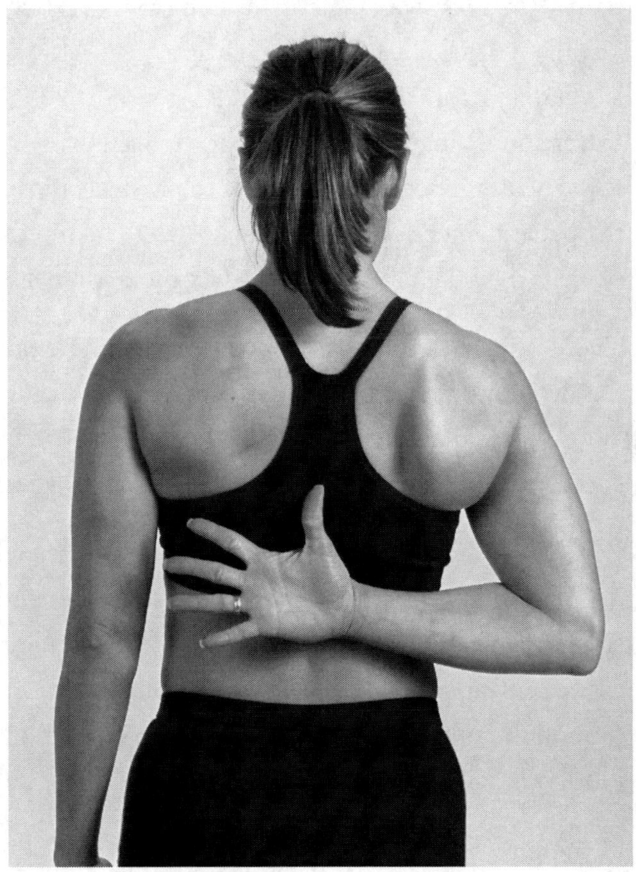

Figure 2.7. Apley ScratchTest (lower).

The Apley's scratch maneuvers are particularly useful in determining an initial baseline, and monitoring progress during treatment such as OMT, and/or physical therapy/rehabilitation of the shoulder.

Neurovascular Examination

Sensorium: Sensation is tested in each dermatome by pinprick and followed by a small brush. The two-point discrimination test is also helpful. A pinwheel is a useful tool to assess pinprick sensation of large areas or along dermatomes or myotomes.

Reflexes:

1. Biceps: The examiner places his or her thumb on the insertion of the biceps tendon. Using a small hammer, the examiner then strikes the thumb.
2. Triceps: The patient's arm is at 90

degrees of vertical abduction and the elbow is flexed to 90 degrees with 90 degrees of internal rotation. The examiner then holds the upper arm in one hand and taps the triceps tendon, which provokes elbow extension. Asymmetry of the amplitude of the reflexes is noted.

NOTE: The brachial plexus traverses the glenohumeral joint on its way down the arm, and shoulder pain can emanate from any plexopathy. Any neurologic deficit can cause pain radiating down the nerves themselves, or create muscle weakness that can lead to shoulder pathology such as rotator cuff impingement and/or scapulothoracic dysfunction. These nerves can be tested through manual muscle testing.

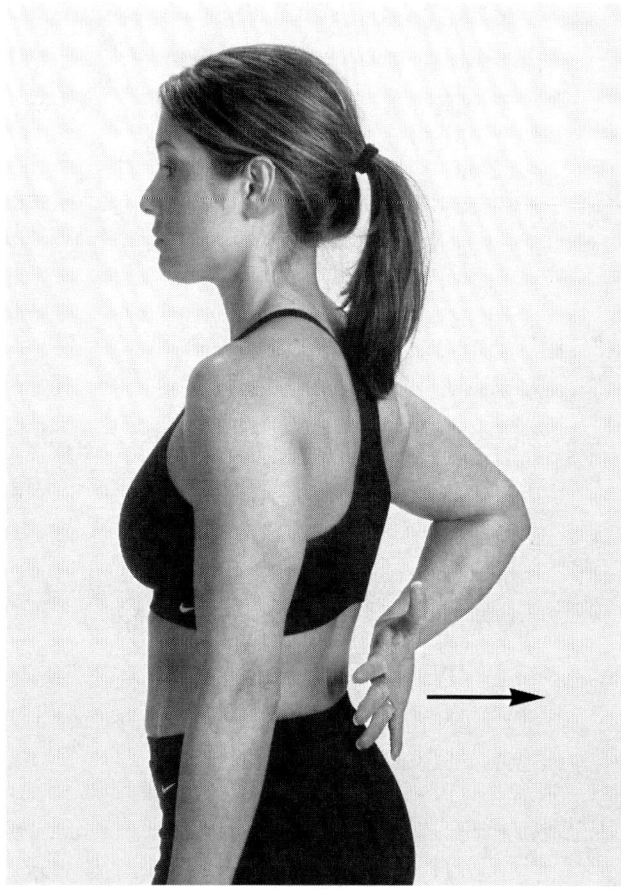

Figure 2.8. Liftoff Test.

Manual Muscle Testing

The list below demonstrates the maneuvers used to test specific muscles for strength. When possible, test bilaterally and simultaneously to detect subtle strength differences.

Specific Strength Testing:

- Deltoid (C5 and C6 - axillary nerve):
  - Anterior deltoid: arm at 90 degrees of abduction, full external rotation and supination. (Alternately, the arm can be at 90 degrees of abduction, palm down, and at 30 degrees of horizontal flexion/adduction.) The examiner provides downward pressure and the patient attempts to raise arm upward.
  - Middle deltoid: arm as for anterior

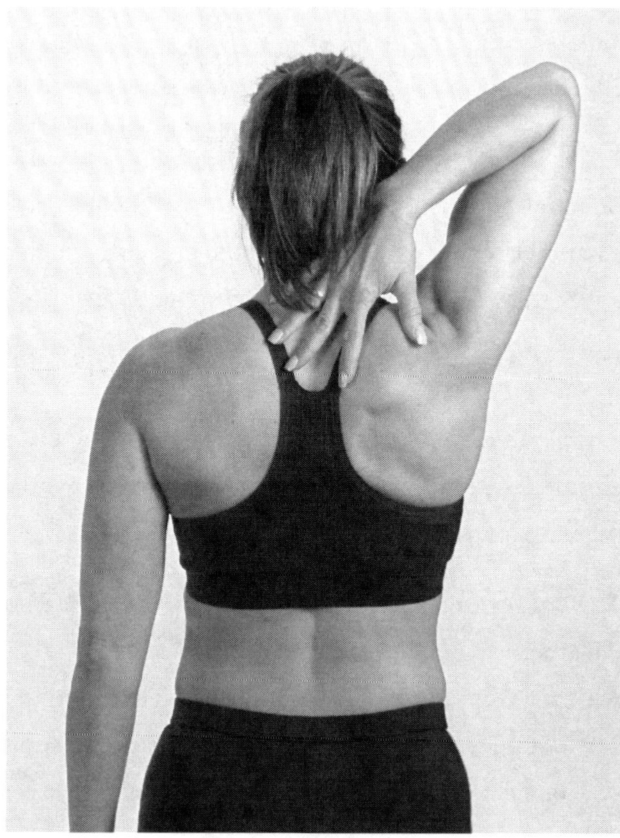

Figure 2.9. Apley Scratch Test (upper).

- deltoid, but with some internal rotation and palm facing down. Again use downward pressure as patient actively elevates the arm.
- Posterior deltoid: arm as for anterior deltoid, but with full internal rotation and palm facing backward. (Alternately, the arm can be at 90 degrees abduction, palm down, and at 30 degrees of horizontal extension.) Resistance applied as above.

- Teres minor: arm at side, elbow at 90 degrees of flexion, patient externally rotates forearm against resistance.
- Infraspinatus: arm at 90 degrees of abduction, elbow partially bent, and resistance applied downward on forearm. Note: This can also be tested with arm at side like teres minor, but we suggest both ways to better detect partial tears.
- Subscapularis: arm at 90 degrees of abduction, resistance directed inward toward the midline.
- Supraspinatus: empty can and/or full can test.
- Trapezius: shrug shoulders against inferior resistance.
- Serratus anterior: arm flexed 90 degrees, palm down, resistance downward.
- Rhomboids: hand on hip with elbow at 90 degrees, resistance anterior against elbow (patient pushes elbows backward).

Supraspinatus (C4-C6, Suprascapular Nerve): Set up patient with arms abducted 90 degrees and adducted 30-45 degrees with the thumbs up (full can test). If the arm does not drop, the examiner can assess strength by the patient's resistance against inferior directed force.

Subscapularis (C5-C7, Upper and Lower Subscapular Nerve): The patient rests the arms at the side with elbows flexed at 90 degrees. The examiner places his or her hands on the ventral aspect of the patient's wrist to resist internal rotation.

Infraspinatus (C5-6, Suprascapular Nerve): The patient sets up as for the subscapularis, and the examiner resists external rotation by placing the hands on the dorsal aspect of the wrist, grading strength (+1 to +5) and noting any elicited pain.

Teres Minor (C5-6, Suprascapular Nerve): Same as for infraspinatus.

Levator Scapulae (C5, Dorsal Scapula Nerve; C3-4, Cervical): Either sitting or standing, the patient elevates the scapula while the examiner resists with the hands on top of the shoulder, pushing inferiorly.

Serratus Anterior (C5-C7, Long Thoracic Nerve): Use the wall push-up test for scapular winging. Another way to test scapulothoracic strength is to ask the patient to put both hands on the hips with the examiner behind him or her. The examiner then offers pressure to the medial aspect of the elbow and asks the patient to push the elbows together posteriorly against the examiner's resistance, noting weakness or scapular winging.

PROVOCATIVE TESTS AND MANEUVERS

Cervical Spine

Pathology emanating from the cervical spine must be ruled out when evaluating shoulder pain / paresthesias.

Spurling's Test. This is the first test to perform when evaluating the cervical intervertebral discs/nerve roots as a source of shoulder pain. The examiner extends the patient's neck and rotates it to one side with corresponding axial compression on the patient's head (see Figure 1.9).

Positive Test: Pain elicited down the ipsilateral arm from the neck.

Indicates: Cervical disc disease/nerve root irritation.

NOTE: Pain produced in the cervical spine ipsilaterally with this maneuver, could suggest facet pathology.

Adson's Test. (See Figure 1.10.) Shoulder pain/tingling could represent thoracic outlet syndrome and this should be ruled out. This test evaluates the subclavian artery for compression by the scalene muscles or a cervical rib.

1. The examiner palpates the radial pulse on the symptomatic arm with the patient's arm at rest.
2. As the pulse is monitored, the examiner moves the patient's arm into 90 degrees abduction and 90 degrees external rotation.
3. The patient takes a deep breath and turns his/her head toward the raised arm.

Positive Test: Marked diminution or loss of pulse/reproduction of patient's symptoms.

Indicates: Subclavian artery compression (vascular, not neurological etiology).

NOTE: Medical students should master at least one of the following provocative tests and each basic test in each category. Residents and physicians should master them all. The basic exam that should be performed on each shoulder exam will be noted accordingly below.

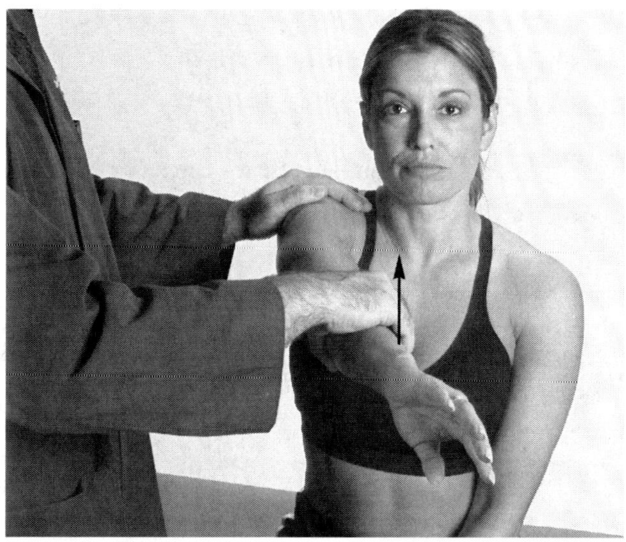

Figure 2.10. Active Compression Test, part I.

Acromioclavicular Joint

Cross-arm Test (Cross-arm Adduction Test) - BASIC EXAM. The examiner passively adducts the patient's arm across the chest wall with the humerus parallel to the floor so that the free hand of the examined elbow rests on the opposite shoulder.

Positive Test: Pain in A-C joint with end-range adduction.

Indicates: Acromioclavicular joint pathology.

Active Compression Test. The patient vertically abducts the arm to 90 degrees and adducts 10 to 15 degrees with internal rotation (thumbs down) (Figure 2.10). The patient resists the examiner's downward force. This maneuver is then repeated with the arm supinated (Figure 2.11).

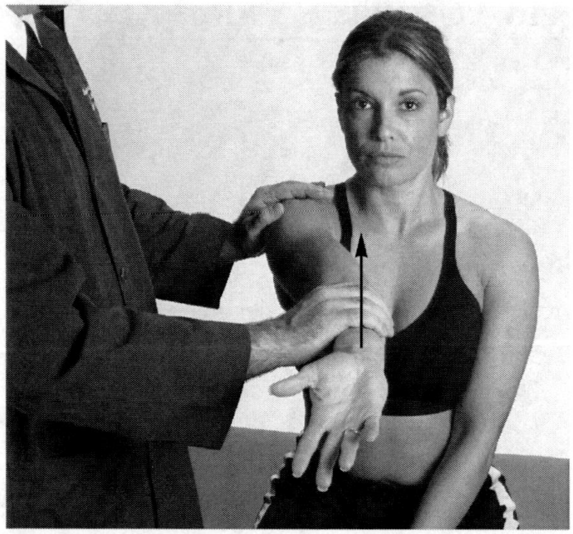

Figure 2.11. Active Compression Test, part II.

Positive Test: Pain that improves or resolves with the second maneuver.

Indicates: Acromioclavicular (AC) pathology if the pain is in the AC joint (or labral pathology if the pain feels more internal in the shoulder).

Scapulothoracic Motion - BASIC EXAM

Range of Motion. The examiner observes scapular rhythm as the patient actively abducts the arms over the head. Note any difference between the scapulae in elevation and depression, external and internal rotation, retraction, and protraction.

Scapular Winging. This is often related to weakness of the serratus anterior, which is innervated by the long thoracic nerve.

Test 1: The patient forward flexes the arms at 90 degrees against clinician's resistance.

Test 2: The patient stands in a relaxed position. Have the patient hang the arms at the side with palms facing backward, then bring them up to a wall or door and perform a push-up off the wall. Observe the scapular behavior (Figure 2.12).

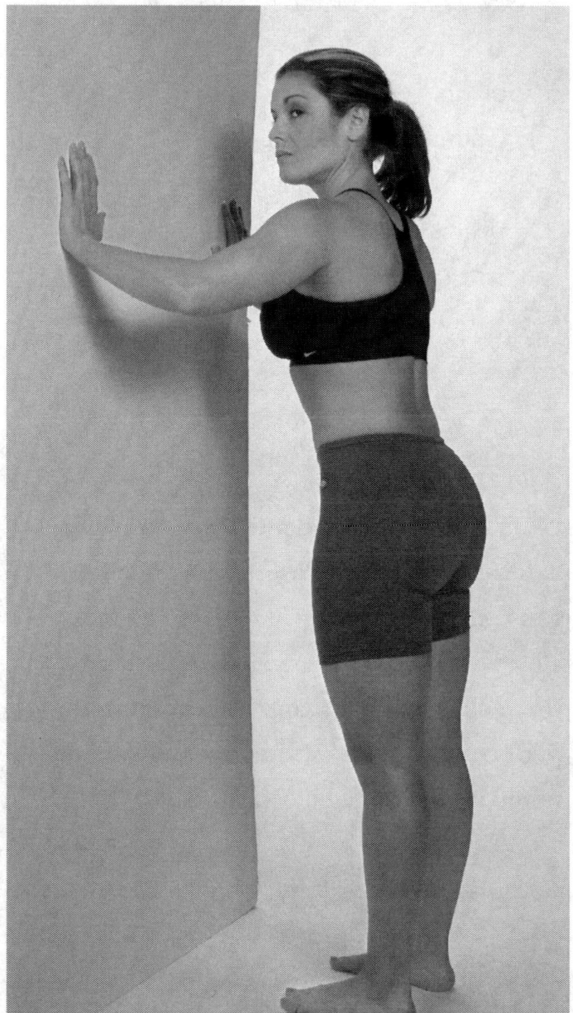

Figure 2.12. Wall pushup to assess scapular winging.

Bicipital Tendon

Speed's Test - BASIC EXAM. This test looks for bicipital groove pathology. The patient's shoulder is in 90 degrees of forward flexion (adduction), elbow extended and hand supinated. Examiner applies resistance to cephalad motion (Figure 2.13).

Positive Test: Pain in the bicipital groove.

Indicates: Bicipital tendon pathology, usually tendinitis.

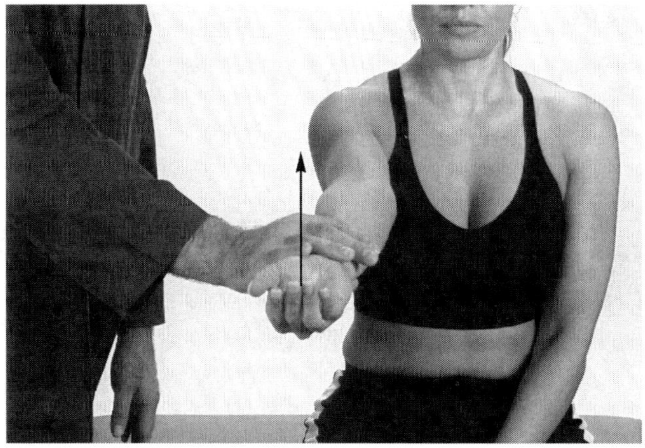

Figure 2.13. Speed's Test.

Yergason's Test. The patient is in the seated position with the elbow at his or her side and flexed to 90 degrees. The examiner palpates the biceps tendon in the bicipital groove with one hand while holding the wrist with the other hand. The examiner then tests the stability of the biceps tendon by having the patient attempt to supinate and externally rotate their forearm against resistance (Figure 2.14).

Positive Test: Tendon will sublux out of groove and/or cause significant pain.

Indicates: Unstable bicipital tendon/ subluxation, subscapularis damage, bicipital tendinitis.

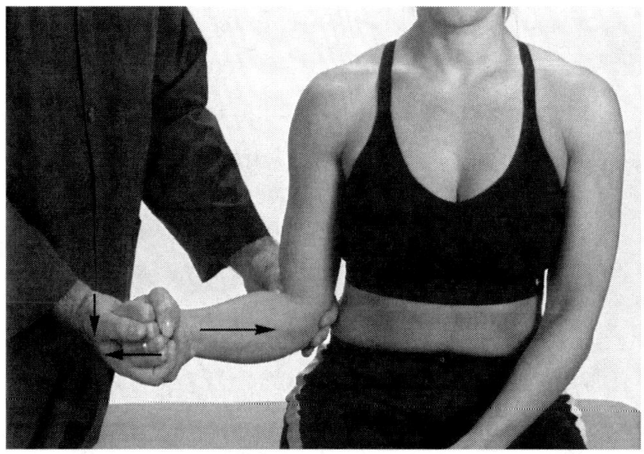

Figure 2.14. Yergason's Test.

Rotator Cuff Testing

Drop Arm Test - BASIC EXAM. The patient elevates both arms into full vertical abduction and then slowly lowers the arms to 90 degrees and holds them in this position

Positive Test: Affected arm will drop to patient's side or a gentle downward tap on the wrist will cause the arm to drop.

Indicates: Full thickness tear of the supraspinatus.

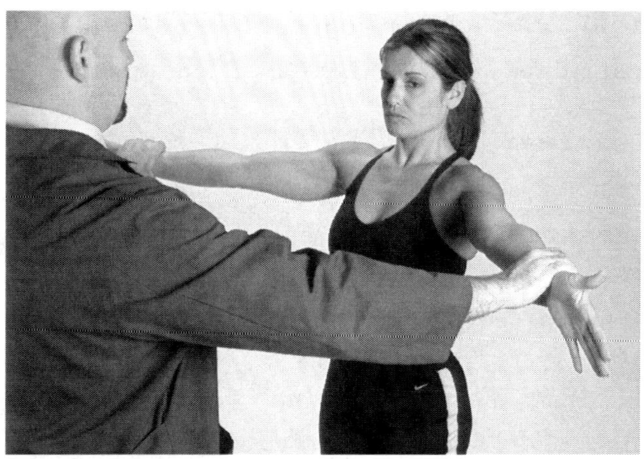

Figure 2.15. Full Can Test.

Full Can Test - BASIC EXAM. The patient abducts both arms to 90 degrees and forward flexes 30-45 degrees with the thumb pointing to the ceiling (Figure 2.15). The patient resists downward pressure.

Positive Test: Weakness or pain.

Indicates: Supraspinatus tendon tear or tendinitis.

NOTE: Recent studies suggest that the full can test is more sensitive for supraspinatus pathology that the empty can test, which has been the standard for years.

Empty Can Test. This test is performed the same as the full can test, but with thumbs down (Figure 2.16).

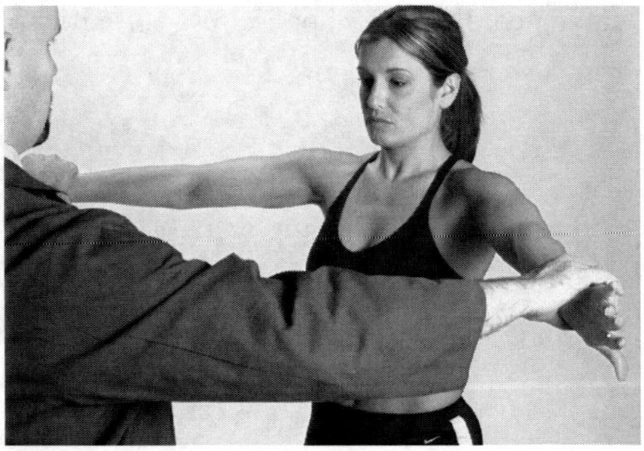

Figure 2.16. Empty Can Test.

Impingement

Painful Arc - BASIC EXAM. The patient abducts the arms overhead as far as they can go, bringing them out laterally (Figure 2.17).

Positive Test: Pain with shoulder abduction between 80 to 100 degrees in the coronal plane.

Indicates: Subacromial impingement.

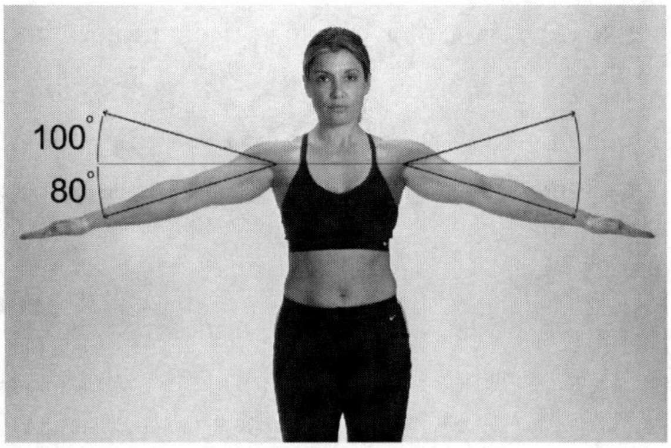

Figure 2.17. Painful Arc.

NOTE: Pain starting after 100 degrees of abduction often suggests acromioclavicular joint pathology; while pain immediately with abduction may indicate adhesive capsulitis, shoulder trauma, or neurapraxia.

Neer Impingement Test - BASIC EXAM. The examiner stabilizes the patient's shoulder on the top with his or her hand, and then passively forward flexes the arm above shoulder level to a full forward flexed position (Figure 2.18).

Positive Test: Provokes pain.

Indicates: Rotator cuff impingement pathology. If pain is provoked with forward flexion to 90 degrees, it is primary impingement.

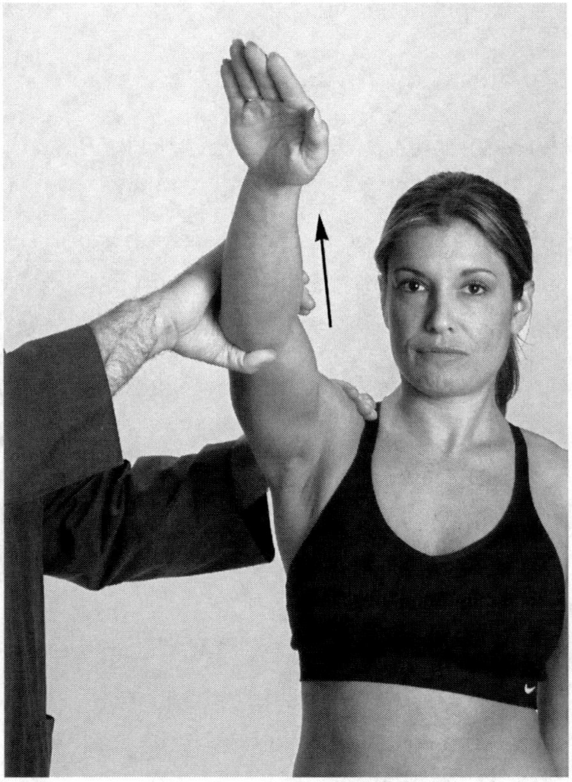

Figure 2.18. Neer Impingement Test.

Hawkins Test (Coracoid Impingement Test). The examiner passively rotates the humerus into internal rotation while forward flexing (adducting) to 90 degrees in the sagittal plane. This opposes the rotator cuff against the coracoacromial ligament and acromion (Figure 2.19).

Positive Test: The maneuver produces pain.

Indicates: Rotator cuff pathology (usually supraspinatus).

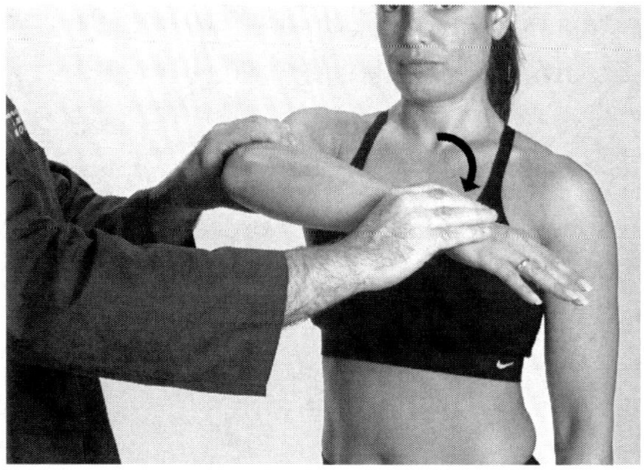

Figure 2.19. Hawkins Test.

Injection Test. The examiner injects the subacromial space with 1% Lidocaine (approximately 5-10ml) and then repeats the impingement test (either Neer's or Hawkin's). If no pain is produced, the examiner knows that the problem is in the subacromial area.

Subscapularis Injury

Gerber's (Liftoff) Test - BASIC EXAM. This evaluates subscapularis muscle strength by limiting pectoralis major firing. The patient puts his or her hand behind the lumbar spine and attempts to lift the hand away from the back (see Figure 2.8).

Positive Test: The patient cannot accomplish the liftoff.

Indicates: Subscapularis injury or weakness.

Napoleon Sign. If the patient cannot fully internally rotate, place the patient's hand on his or her stomach and have the patient push against it (Figure 2.20).

Positive Test: The elbow will drop backward.

Indicates: Subscapularis injury or weakness.

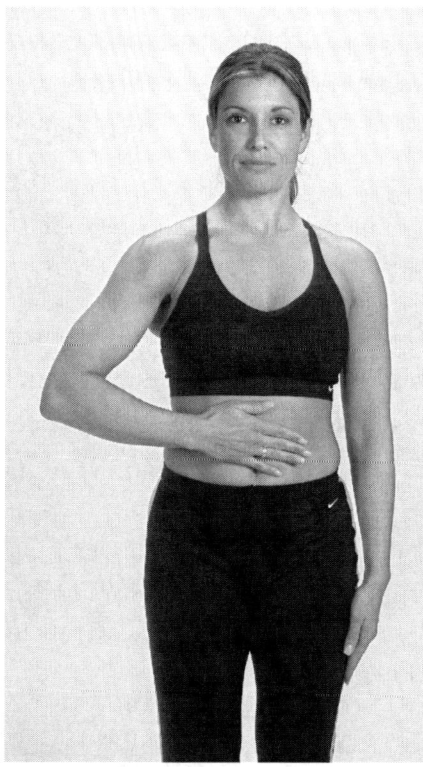

Figure 2.20. Napoleon Sign.

Glenohumeral Instability/Labral Pathology (these often occur together)

Sulcus Sign - BASIC EXAM. The patient's elbow is grasped and inferior traction is applied.

Positive Test: An indentation appears in the area beneath the acromion.

Indicates: Inferior instability, multidirectional instability..

Apprehension Sign (Crank Test) - BASIC EXAM. The patient is in sitting or supine position, with the arm vertically abducted to 90 degrees and the elbow flexed to 90 degrees. The forearm is then forced into external rotation past 90 degrees (Figure 2.21).

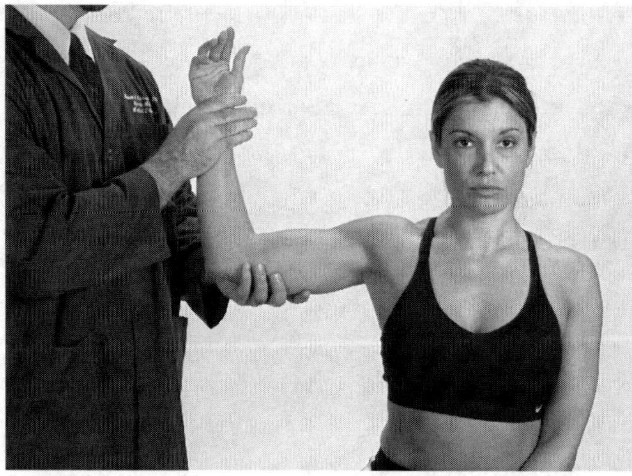

Figure 2.21. Apprehension sign positioning.

Positive Test: The patient will become very apprehensive and ask the examiner to stop for fear of a repeat dislocation.

Indicates: Glenohumeral instability, previous glenohumeral dislocation or subluxation.

Relocation Test. With the patient supine, rotate the arm into abduction and external rotation, similar to the apprehension sign. If the patient feels unstable or apprehensive, the examiner then presses on the anterior aspect of the humerus with other hand toward the table (Figure 2.22). A positive relocation test is an improvement of symptoms. From here, bring the humerus into further external rotation while continuing to stabilize the anterior shoulder. If the patient's shoulder pain becomes worse when the anterior shoulder is suddenly released, this is called a ***Positive Release Test*** or ***Surprise Test*** and corroborates the apprehension sign.

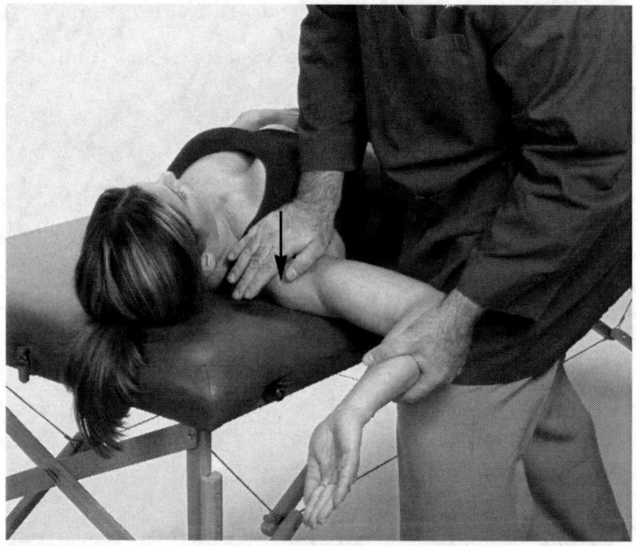

Figure 2.22. Relocation Test.

NOTE: A positive test on the apprehension, relocation, and surprise examinations is highly specific for glenohumeral instability. Additionally, Ian et al.[2] found the surprise test was significantly more specific than the relocation test.1 In fact, the relocation test failed to identify instability in a significant portion of subjects tested.

Clunk Test. The patient is supine, and the examiner's hand is posterior to the humeral head. The examiner applies an anterior force to the humeral head, while the opposite hand holds the distal humerus and rotates it. The patient's arm is then brought overhead into a fully abducted position (Figure 2.23).

Positive Test: A clunk or grinding in the shoulder.

Indicates: Labral pathology.

Active Compression Test (O'Brien's Test) - BASIC EXAM. To perform this test, see the section on Acromioclavicular tests for shoulder complaints: Pain for labral damage is deep inside the glenohumeral joint (see Figure 2.10 and Figure 2.11).

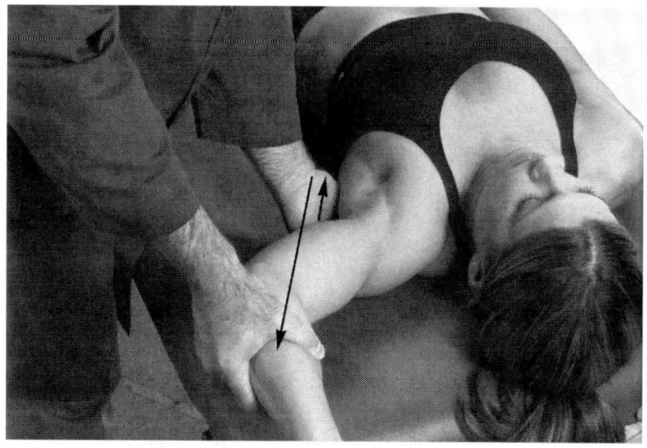

Figure 2.23. Clunk Test.

Positive Test: Pain occurs in the first maneuver but improves or resolves with the second maneuver. Pain is located deep in the shoulder, as opposed to acromioclavicular pathology, which can also cause a positive test, but with pain in AC joint.

Indicates: Labral pathology (if pain is deep inside the shoulder).

NOTE: Now that a clinical diagnosis has been made, the Seven Stages of Spencer can be performed (if appropriate) with corresponding treatment.

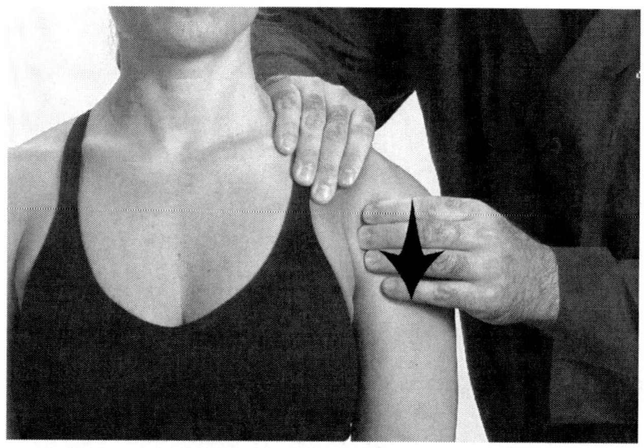

Figure 2.24. Load shift showing compression of humeralhead into glenoid.

Load Shift Test. The examiner stands behind the seated patient and places one hand over the shoulder and scapula to steady the shoulder girdle. The opposite hand grasps the humeral head, fingers upon the medial edge, and pushes it into the glenoid fossa (Figure 2.24). The examiner then shifts the head anteriorly, then posteriorly, noting pain and clicking, and measuring translation in each direction by a +1 to +3 scale. In a +3 load shift the humerus can be subluxed out of the glenohumeral joint.

COMMON CONDITIONS

- Fractures
  - Clavicle
  - Acromion
  - Humeral head
  - Humeral shaft
  - Scapula
- Impingement
  - Bursitis

- Rotator cuff tendonitis/tear
  - AC joint pathology, Osteolysis of AC joint
  - Adhesive capsulitis
  - Labral tears, SLAP tears
  - Nerve impingements
- Muscular Strains
  - Pectoral
  - Biceps
  - Triceps
  - Rotator cuff
    - Supraspinatus
    - Infraspinatus
    - Subscapularis
    - Teres Minor
- Biceps Tendinitis
- Osteoarthiritis
- A-C Sprains
- Glenohumeral Dislocations/Subluxations

CONDITIONS THAT SHOULD NOT BE MISSED DUE TO MORBIDITY OR MORTALITY

- Fractures (See above)
  - epiphyseal
  - anatomic neck
  - greater tuberosity
  - surgical neck fractures of the humerus
- Dislocations
- Tumors
- Neurologic injury (contusion/laceration) causing neurapraxia/paralysis

REFERENCES

1. Trumble TE, Budoff JE, Cornwell R. *Hand, Elbow, and Shoulder: Core Knowledge in Orthopedics.* Mosby, Inc.; 2006:557.
2. Ian KY, Lo IKY, Nonweiler B, et al. *An evaluation of the apprehension, relocation, and surprise tests for anterior shoulder instability.* Am J Sports Medicine. 2004; 32:301-307.
3. Karageanes SJ. *Principles of Manual Sports Medicine.* Philadelphia, PA: Lippincott Williams & Wilkins; 2005.

3 The Elbow Joint Exam

Anna L. Avik, D.O., ATC, PGYI, Orthopedic Surgery Resident

Thomas Wesley Allen, D.O., FCCP, FACOI, FACP, FAOASM

Kim Grillo, D.O., PGYI, Orthopedic Surgery Resident

Jason Tarno, D.O., FAOASM

Phillip Zinni III, D.O., FAOASM, CMRO, MS, ATC

ANATOMY

The elbow is a hinge joint between the humerus, radius, and ulna, and is surrounded by a fibrous capsule. Articulations exist between these three bones to allow the motions of flexion and extension about the joint.

Bones

Humerus: The distal end of the humerus broadens to form the medial and lateral epicondyles and one central condyle. The medial and lateral epicondyles serve as attachment sites for the flexor and extensor muscular compartments of the forearm, respectively. The posterior aspect of the medial epicondyle also contains the ulnar groove, or cubital tunnel, which houses the ulnar nerve. The lateral condyle articulates with the capitulum and the medial condyle articulates with the trochlea.

Radius: The proximal end of the radius consists of the oval shaped radial head, radial neck, and radial tuberosity. The radial tuberosity lies medially and just inferior to the neck, and serves as the insertion site for the biceps brachii muscle.

Ulna: The proximal end of the ulna contains the olecranon posteriorly, coronoid process anteriorly, radial notch laterally, and trochlear notch centrally. The olecranon serves as the attachment site for the triceps brachii muscle, and is palpable as the 'tip' of the elbow. The troclear notch is the large depression lying between the olecranon and coronoid process.

Articulations

The trochlea of the humerus articulates with the trochlear notch of the ulna forming the humeroulnar joint, and the capitulum of the humerus articulates with the radial head forming the humeroradial joint. Flexion and extension at the elbow are permitted by the humeroulnar joint and to a lesser degree the humeroradial joint. The humeroulnar joint also prevents abnormal or excessive hyperextension or dislocation at the joint.

The radial head articulates with the radial notch of the ulna to form the radioulnar joint. This joint is responsible for rotation of the radius about the elbow joint, allowing pronation and supination of the forearm.

Pads of fat lie over both the coronoid fossa and olecranon fossa. These fat pads serve as cushions within the joint, and are moved out of impingement areas during flexion and extension by the insertions of the brachialis and triceps brachii. The posterior fat pad may become engorged with blood during an acute intra-articular hemorrhage.

NOTE: On lateral radiograph of the arm with the elbow in ninety degrees flexion, this is

seen as an area of lucency behind the olecranon. This finding is called the posterior fat pad sign and is indicative of an occult fracture.

Ligaments

The fibrous capsule of the elbow joint is thickened medially and laterally to form the medial and lateral collateral ligaments. These ligaments aid in support during flexion and extension movements of the joint.

The medial collateral ligament contains anterior, posterior, and oblique bands. The anterior band is the most important medial stabilizer, coursing from the medial epicondyle proximally to the coronoid process distally. The posterior band attaches from the medial epicondyle to the olecranon process, and the oblique band attaches from the olecranon to the coronoid process.

The lateral collateral ligament is reinforced by the annular ligament of the radius. The annular ligament surrounds the head of the radius and stabilizes supination and pronation or the forearm.

Cubital Fossa

The cubital fossa is a triangular depression lying anterior to the elbow joint and contains from lateral to medial the biceps brachii tendon, the brachial artery, and the median nerve. The base of the fossa is a line between the medial and lateral epicondyles, and the lateral and medial borders are formed by the brachioradialis muscle and pronator teres muscle, respectively. The median cubital vein courses across the cubital tunnel as it connects the medial basilic vein to the lateral cephalic vein.

Vascular Supply

The brachial artery courses superficial to the elbow joint through the cubital fossa and divides into the radial and ulnar arteries at the level of the radial head. Collateral and recurrent branches of the brachial, radial, ulnar, and profunda brachii arteries supply the elbow joint.

Innervation

The musculocutaneous, median, ulnar, and radial nerves contribute to innervation about the elbow joint. The biceps brachii and brachialis muscles are innervated by the musculocutaneous nerve. All muscles in the anterior compartment of the forearm are innervated by the median nerve, except for the flexor carpi ulnaris and medial half of the flexor digitorum profundus, which are innervated by the ulnar nerve. All muscles in the posterior compartment of the forearm along with the triceps brachii and brachioradialis muscles are innervated by the radial nerve (Table 3.1).

Table 3.1. Muscles Surrounding the Elbow Joint

Muscle	Origin	Insertion	Innervation	Action
Biceps brachii	Short head-coracoid process, long head-supraglenoid tubercle of scapula	Radial tuberosity	Musculocutaneous nerve	Flexes forearm when supinated, supinates forearm
Coracobrachialis	Coracoid process	Medial surface and border of humerus	Musculocutaneous nerve	Flexes and adducts arm
Brachialis	Distal half of anterior humerus	Tuberosity and coronoid process of ulna	Musculocutaneous nerve	Flexes forearm
Brachioradialis	Lateral supracondylar ridge of humerus	Lateral distal radius	Radial nerve	Flexes forearm
Triceps brachii	Infraglenoid tubercle of scapula, posterior surface of humerus	Posterior portion of proximal olecranon	Radial nerve	Extends forearm
Anconeus	Lateral epicondyle of humerus	Lateral olecranon, body of ulna	Radial nerve	Extends forearm, abducts ulna during pronation
Pronator teres	Medial epicondyle, intermuscular septum, coronoid process	Midway along lateral surface of radius	Median nerve	Pronates and flexes forearm
Pronator quadratus	Distal ulna, medial side	Lateral border of distal radius, volar side	Median nerve	Pronates forearm
Flexor carpi radialis	Medial epicondyle of humerus	2nd and 3rd metacarpal bones	Median nerve	Flexes and abducts hand
Palmaris longus	Medial epicondyle	Flexor retinaculum and palmar aponeurosis	Median nerve	Flexes hand
Flexor carpi ulnaris	Medial epicondyle and olecranon	Pisiform bone, hook of hamate, 5th metacarpal	Ulnar nerve	Flexes and adducts hand
Flexor digitorum superficialis	Medial epicondyle of humerus, coronoid process, anterior radius	Middle phalanges digits 2-5	Median nerve	Flexes middle phalanges at PIP joints, flexes proximal phalanges at MCP joints
Flexor digitorum profundus	Proximal ulna, volar side	Distal phalanges digits 2-5	Medial half of FDP --ulnar nerve; lateral half of FDP -- anterior interosseus branch of the median nerve	Flexes distal phalanges at DIP joints, assists w flexion at PIP and MP joints
Flexor pollicis longus	Anterior radius	Base of distal phalanx of thumb	Median nerve	Flexes proximal phalanx and distal phalanx of thumb

Table 3.1. Muscles Surrounding the Elbow Joint (Continued)

Muscle	Origin	Insertion	Innervation	Action
Supinator	Lateral epicondyle of humerus, proximal radioulnar joint	Proximal radius	Deep branch of radial nerve	Supinates forearm
Extensor carpi radialis longus	Lateral supracondylar ridge of humerus	Base of the 2nd metacarpal	Radial nerve	Extends and abducts hand
Extensor carpi radialis brevis	Lateral epicondyle of humerus	Base of the 3rd metacarpal bone	Deep branch of radial nerve	Extends and abducts hand
Extensor digitorum	Lateral epicondyle of humerus	Extensor expansions of medial 4 digits	Deep branch of radial nerve (posterior interosseous nerve)	Extends digits at MCP and IP joints, extends hand
Extensor digiti minimi	Lateral epicondyle of humerus	Extensor expansion of fifth digit	Deep branch of radial nerve (posterior interosseous nerve)	Extends 5th digit at MCP and IP joints
Extensor carpi ulnaris	Lateral epicondyle of humerus, dorsal ulna	Base of 5th metacarpal bone	Deep branch of radial nerve (posterior interosseous nerve)	Extends and adducts hand
Abductor pollicis longus	Dorsal radius and ulna	Base of 1st metacarpal bone	Deep branch of radial nerve (posterior interosseous nerve)	Abducts thumb
Extensor pollicis brevis	Dorsal radius	Base of proximal phalanx of thumb	Deep branch of radial nerve (posterior interosseous nerve)	Extends proximal phalanx of thumb
Extensor pollicis longus	Dorsal ulna	Base of distal phalanx of thumb	Deep branch of radial nerve (posterior interosseous nerve)	Extends distal phalanx of thumb
Extensor indicis	Dorsal ulna	Extensor expansion of index finger	Deep branch of radial nerve (posterior interosseous nerve)	Extends index finger

PHYSICAL EXAM

Elbow pain can be from an acute injury such as falling on an outstretched hand, or from chronic overuse such as in a throwing athlete. In a suspected acute injury, history should include questions about position of the elbow joint during injury, the direction and amount of force applied, and whether a 'pop' was felt or heard. With chronic injuries, we must determine what specific movements cause pain. For example, in a baseball player, identify which phase of the pitching motion reproduces pain. Further, history of catching or locking within the joint and numbness or tingling surrounding the joint must be noted.

Observation

Look at both elbows to compare any apparent skin or muscle changes, including erythema, scars, swelling, or atrophy. Distinguish generalized swelling of the elbow and surrounding tissues from localized swelling at a specific location, such as around the olecranon process. Also, pay close attention to excessive skin irritation, heat, or erythema, as these characteristics may represent a more serious injury, or infection.

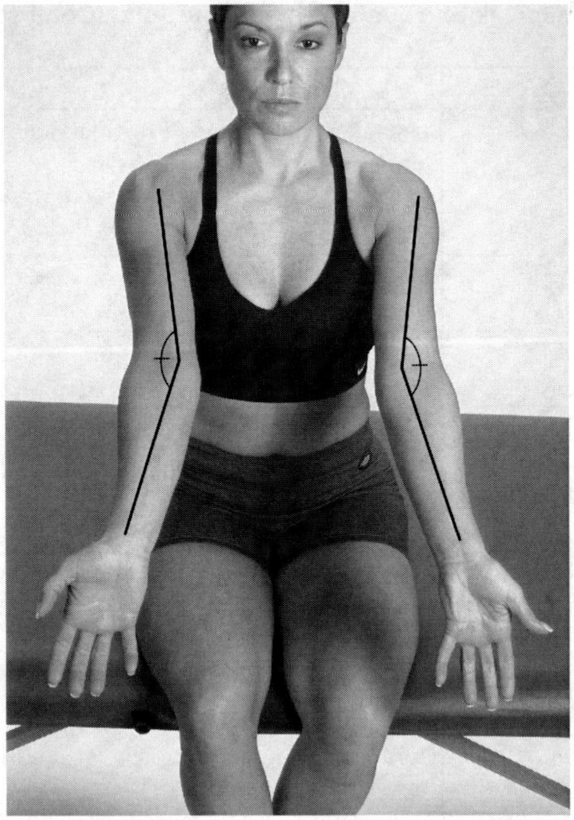

Figure 3.1. Carrying angle of the elbow.

Compare both elbows for alignment and carrying angle and note any abnormal angulation. The carrying angle is a lateral or valgus angle formed by the intersection of a line through the center of the humerus, and one through the center of the forearm (Figure 3.1). A normal carrying angle measures between 5 and 10 degrees, and may be up to 5 degrees greater in women.

Alignment is also measured by comparing the epicondyles in relation to the olecranon with the elbow at ninety degrees of flexion. There should be equidistance between the epicondyles and olecranon, and the olecranon should lie in line with the center of the humeral shaft. If not, a fracture or dislocation could be present.

Palpation

The medial epicondyle is palpated as the bony structure at the medial portion of the elbow joint (Figure 3.2). Several muscles that flex the wrist and fingers, and pronate the hand share a common origin at the medial epicondyle.

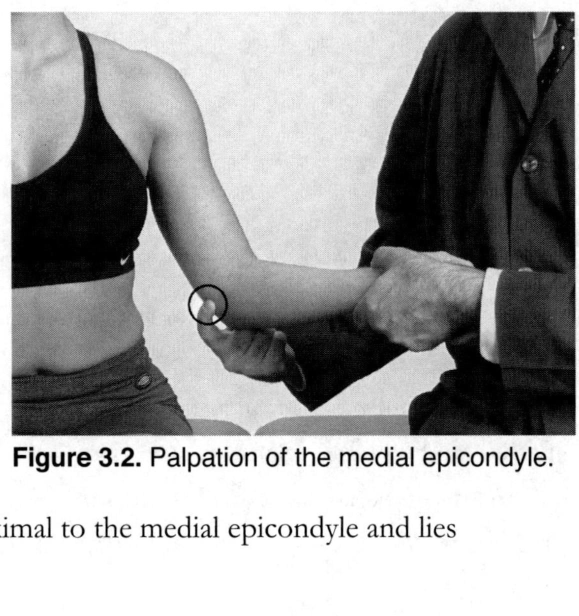

Figure 3.2. Palpation of the medial epicondyle.

The medial supracondylar region of the humerus is palpated just proximal to the medial epicondyle. The supracondylar landmark is often used when describing location of a fracture or other injury.

The medial collateral ligament originates just proximal to the medial epicondyle and lies over the medial compartment of the elbow joint. Palpate this ligament from its origin distally to the ulna, assessing for tenderness, bogginess, or irregularity (Figure 3.3). Note that the flexor carpi ulnaris muscle lies above the medial collateral ligament and tenderness in this area may not be specific to the medial collateral ligament.

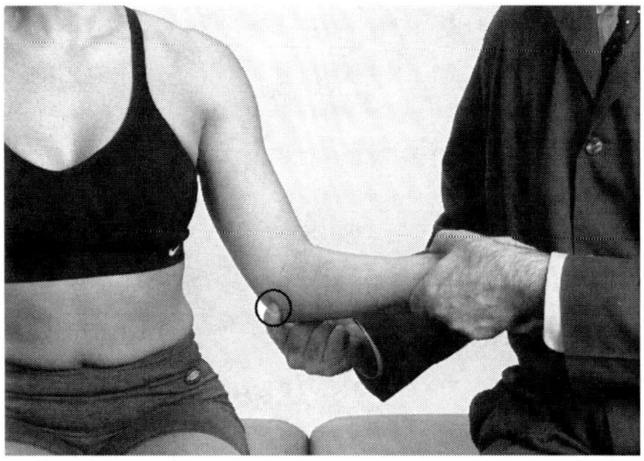

Figure 3.3. Palpation of the medial collateral ligament.

The ulnar nerve passes behind the medial epicondyle and can be palpated in this region against the bone. **NOTE: Pain upon palpation or tapping in this area producing a positive *Tinel's Sign*, may suggest ulnar irritation or neuropathy, known as cubital tunnel syndrome.**

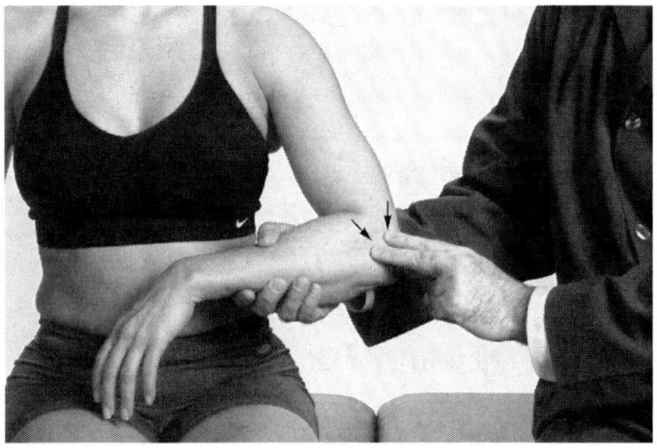

Figure 3.4. Palpation of the lateral epicondyle (index finger), and radial head (middle finger).

Laterally, one can palpate the lateral epicondyle where the distal humerus joins the elbow joint (Figure 3.4). The origin of the supinator muscle and several extensor muscles share a common origin at the lateral epicondyle. The lateral supracondylar region of the humerus is palpated just proximal to the lateral epicondyle.

The radial nerve passes along the lateral supracondylar region from the arm into the posterior forearm, traveling from posterior to anterior compartments. Palpate 3-4 cm distal and just medial to the lateral epicondyle on the dorsal forearm. Tenderness suggests radial nerve entrapment or injury.

The radial head is found just distal to the lateral epicondyle (see Figure 3.4), and is best palpated using the thumb and index finger to surround the structure. Supination and pronation of the forearm is helpful to feel the rotation of the radial head and ensure your location.

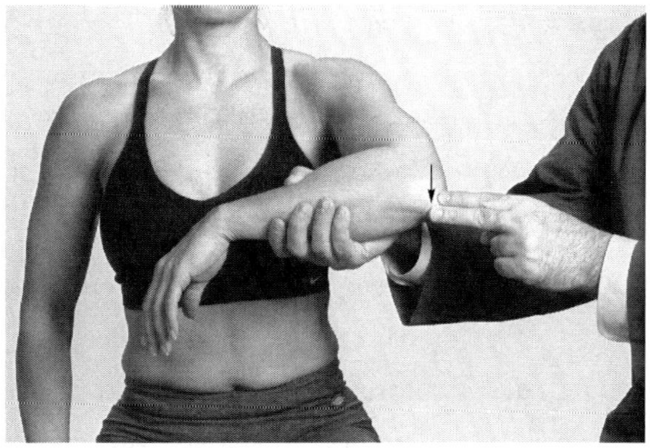

Figure 3.5. Palpation of the olecranon process.

Posteriorly, the olecranon is palpated as the tip of the elbow (Figure 3.5). The triceps tendon inserts at the olecranon and is covered by the olecranon bursa superficially.

Anteriorly, the biceps tendon is located within the cubital fossa and inserts into the radial tuberosity. The brachial artery can also be palpated within the cubital fossa just medial to the biceps tendon.

Range of Motion

Flexion and extension occur primarily about the humeroulnar articulation. Normal flexion is 140 to 150 degrees (Figure 3.6), and normal extension is 0-5 degrees (Figure 3.7).

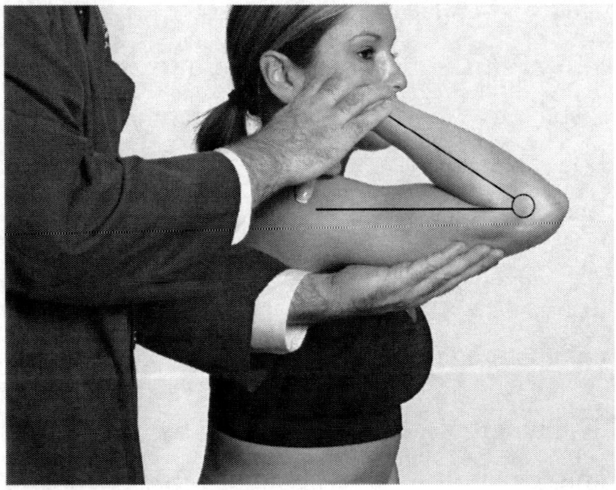

Figure 3.6. Elbow flexion.

Pronation and supination occur primarily about the radioulnar articulation. These motions are best tested beginning with the elbow at 90 degrees flexion and the thumb pointed up. Normal pronation is 90 degrees with the palm facing down (Figure 3.8) and normal supination is 90 degrees with the palm facing up (Figure 3.9).

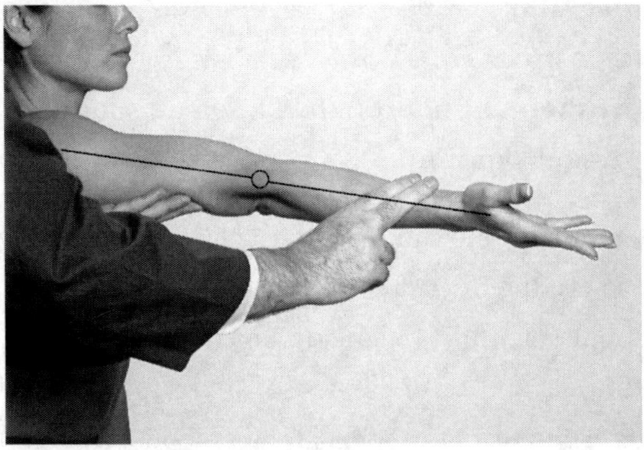

Figure 3.7. Elbow extension.

Pain, restriction (suggesting possible radial head dysfunction), locking or catching within or about the joint during any of these motions should be noted.

Manual Muscle Testing

Triceps: The patient's arm is slightly flexed and the elbow is flexed to 90 degrees. The examiner places one hand under the elbow joint for stabilization and the other hand at the distal forearm to resist the movement. Instruct the patient to extend the forearm.

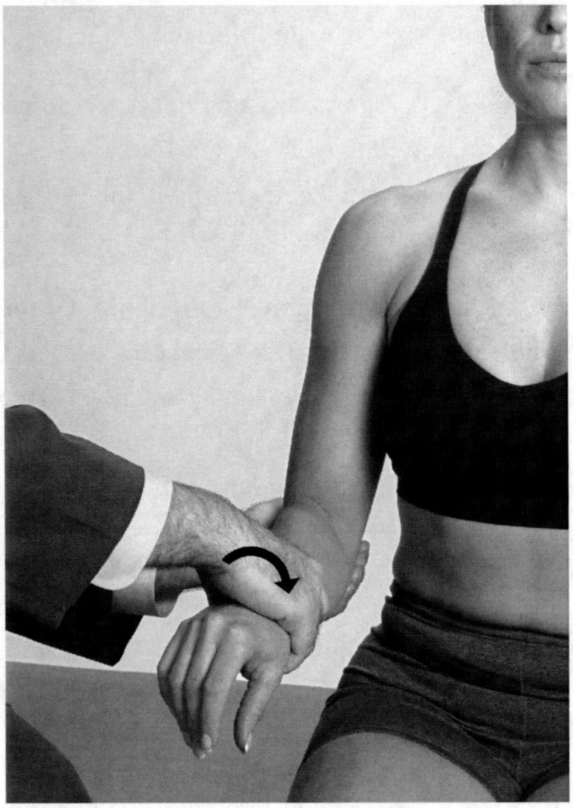

Figure 3.8. Elbow/forearm pronation.

Biceps brachii: The patient's elbow is flexed to 90 degrees and forearm is placed in supination with the palm facing up. The examiner places one hand under elbow for stabilization and the other hand at the distal forearm to resist movement. Instruct the patient to flex the forearm (Figure 3.10). Next, the patient's elbow is flexed to 90 degrees and the forearm is placed in pronation with the palm facing down. The examiner places one hand under the elbow for stabilization and the other hand at the distal forearm to resist movement. Instruct the patient to supinate the forearm.

Brachialis: The patient's elbow is flexed to 90 degrees and forearm is placed in pronation with the palm facing down. The examiner places one hand under elbow for stabilization and the other hand at the distal forearm. Instruct the patient to flex the forearm (Figure 3.11).

Brachioradialis: The patient's elbow is flexed to 90 degrees and forearm is placed in neutral with the palm facing medially. The examiner places one hand under elbow for stabilization and the other hand at the distal forearm. Instruct the patient to flex the forearm.

Anterior/Flexor Forearm Compartment: The patient's elbow is flexed to 90 degrees and forearm is placed in supination with the wrist neutral and palm facing up. The examiner places one hand under the proximal forearm for stabilization and the other hand over the patient's hand to resist movement. Instruct the patient to flex the wrist.

Posterior/Extensor Forearm Compartment: The patient's elbow is flexed to 90 degrees and forearm is placed in pronation with the wrist neutral and palm facing down. The examiner places one hand under the proximal forearm for stabilization and the other hand over the patient's hand to resist movement. Instruct the patient to extend the wrist.

Reflexes

Biceps (C5): With the patient's arm resting on his or her lap, palpate the biceps tendon at its insertion on the radial tuberosity just distal to the cubital fossa. Gently strike the tendon with a reflex hammer. The patient's arm should slightly flex.

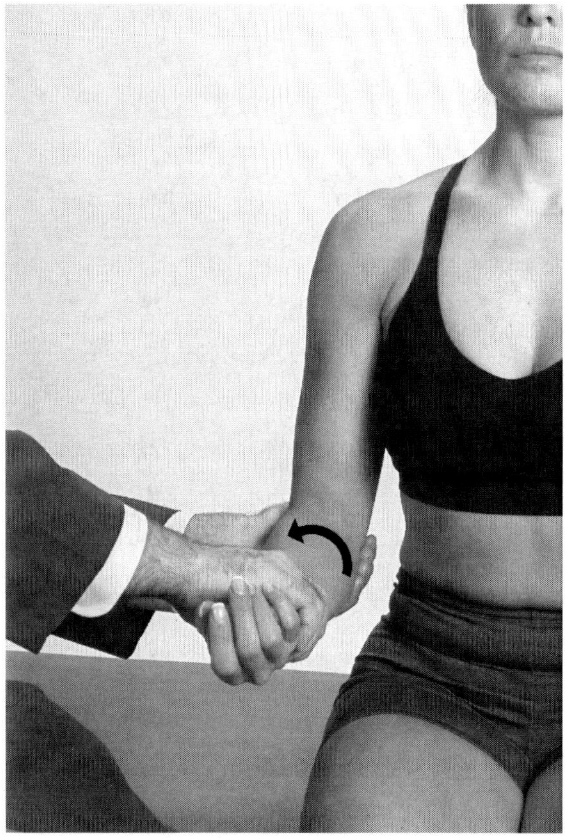

Figure 3.9. Elbow/forearm supination.

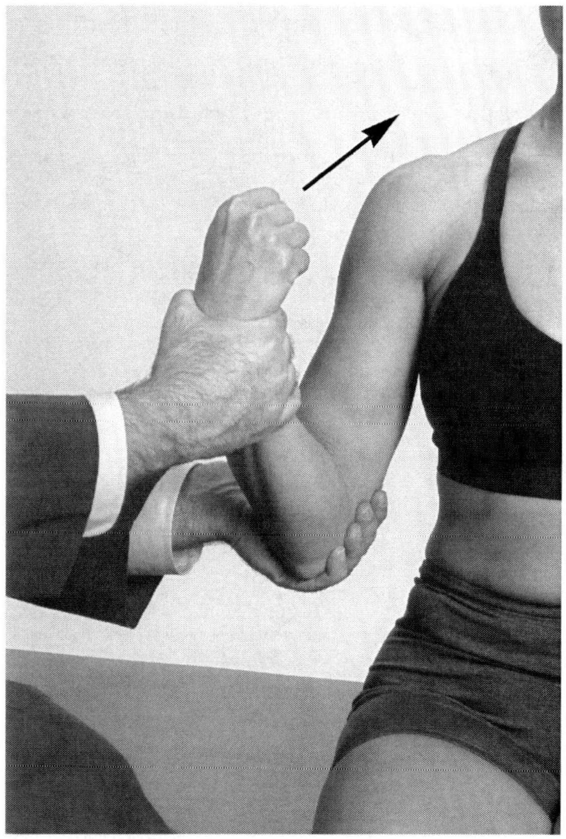

Figure 3.10. Manual muscle testing of the biceps brachii muscle.

Brachioradialis (C6): With the patient's arm resting on his or her lap, palpate the brachioradialis tendon on the distal volar radius about 10cm proximal to the wrist. The wrist should slightly extend as the area is gently tapped with the reflex hammer.

Triceps (C7): Abduct the patient's arm to 90 degrees, with the elbow remaining at 90 degrees flexion, and 90 degrees of internal rotation. Palpate the tendon of the triceps muscle at its insertion on the olecranon and gently strike with a reflex hammer. The elbow should slightly extend.

Sensory

The C5 dermatome courses along the lateral arm and is tested by palpating the lateral epicondyle. The C6 dermatome courses along the radial forearm, thumb, and distal index finger. Sensation of the third finger tests the C7 dermatome, while sensation of the fourth and fifth fingers as well as the hypothenar eminence tests the C8 dermatome. The ulnar forearm and medial epicondyle are within the T1 dermatome.

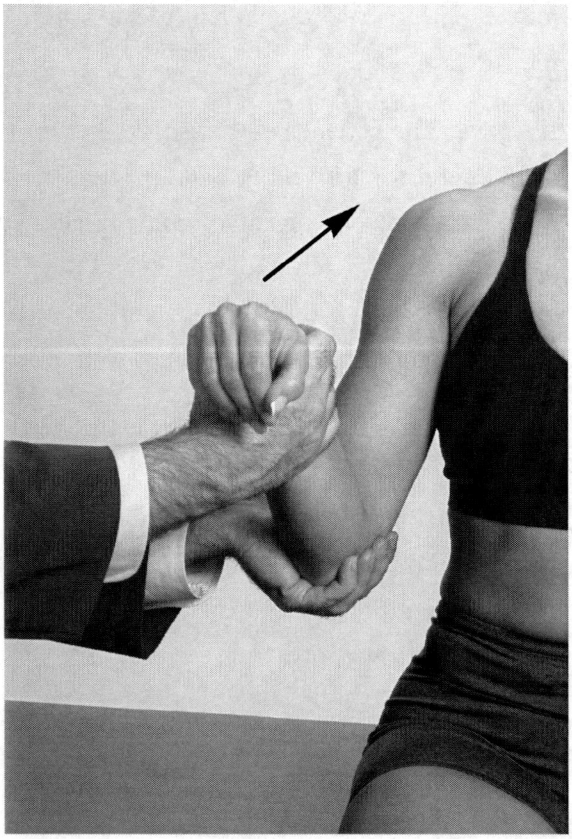

Figure 3.11. Manual muscle testing of the brachialis muscle.

PROVOCATIVE TESTS FOR BASIC EXAM

Medial Collateral Ligament Stability

Valgus Stress Test. The arm is slightly abducted and externally rotated, the forearm is supinated, and the elbow is flexed to 30 degrees. A slight medial directed valgus stress is applied to the elbow joint (Figure 3.12).

Positive Test: Pain or increased laxity as compared with contralateral side.

Indicates: Medial collateral ligament injury.

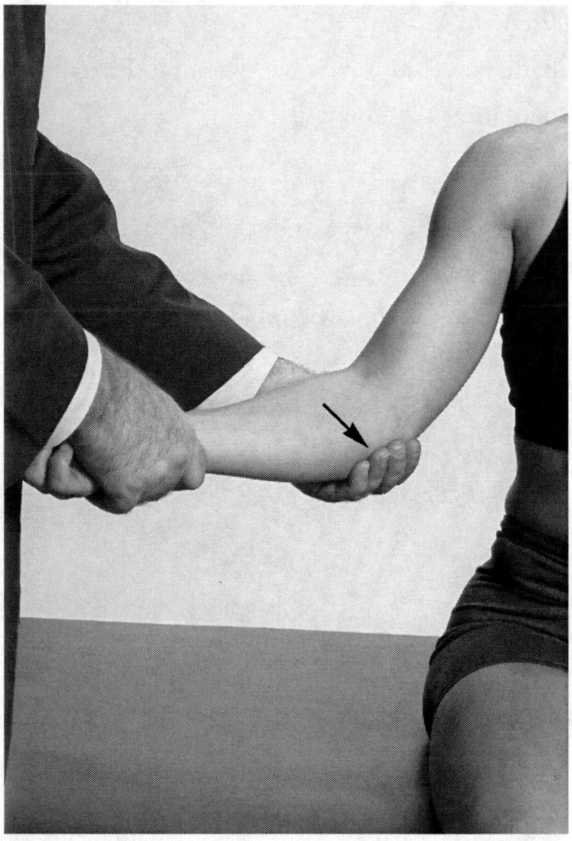

Figure 3.12. Valgus stress of medial collateral ligament with elbow at 30 degrees of flexion.

Lateral Collateral Ligament Stability

Varus Stress Test. The arm is slightly abducted and internally rotated, and elbow flexed to 15 degrees. A slight varus stress is applied to the elbow joint (Figure 3.13).

Positive Test: Pain or increased laxity as compared with contralateral side.

Indicates: Lateral collateral ligament injury.

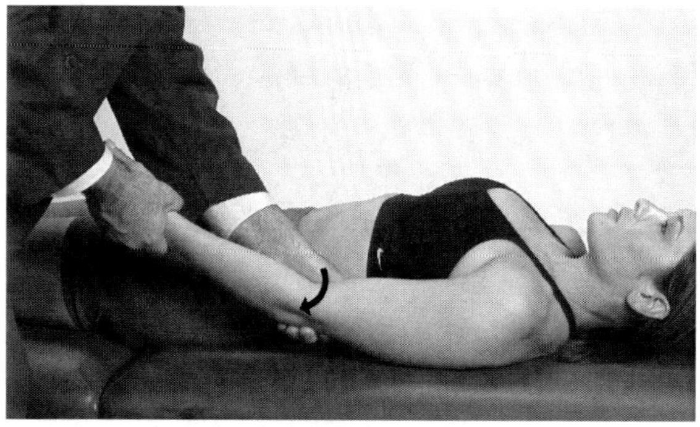

Figure 3.13. Varus stress of lateral collateral ligament with elbow flexed approximately 15 degrees.

Tinel's Sign. The examiner taps between the olecranon and the medial epicondyle in the ulnar groove.

Positive Test: Eliciting a tingling sensation down the forearm within the ulnar nerve distribution.

Indicates: Cubital tunnel syndrome, or ulnar nerve trauma.

Radial Head Instability/Nursemaid's Elbow. The patient usually presents with the elbow slightly pronated, flexed, and held close to the trunk. History most commonly reveals a sudden pull of the arm when the elbow is fully extended. For example, an adult may pull a child's hand or arm upwards to prevent a fall.

Positive Test: Tenderness or pain upon palpation of the anterolateral radial head with usual anterior displacement of the radial head. Posterior glide of the radial head is restricted.

Indicates: Subluxation of the radial head from the annular ligament or somatic dysfunction of the radial head.

Cozen's Test. The patient is sitting with the elbow flexed 90 degrees. The examiner stabilizes the elbow, and instructs the patient to make a fist, pronate and extend the wrist, as the examiner applies a resistive force.

Positive Test: Pain at the lateral epicondyle.

Indicates: Lateral epicondylitis

PROVOCATIVE TESTS FOR COMPLETE EXAM

Milking Sign. The arm is abducted to 90 degrees and the elbow is flexed to 90 degrees. The examiner stabilizes the elbow joint on its radial side with one hand and grasps the

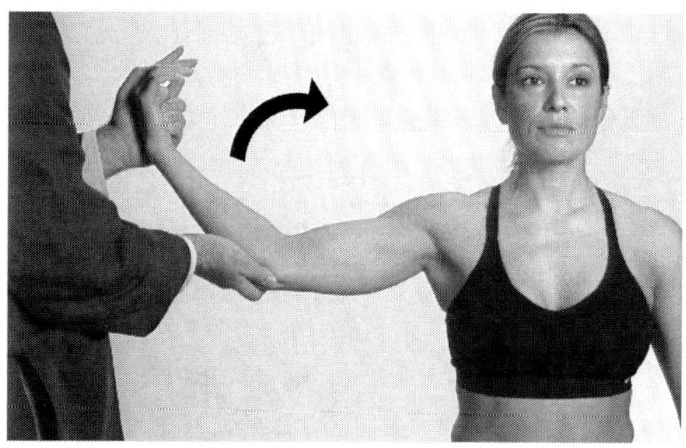

Figure 3.14. Milking Sign.

patients hand with other. The examiner slowly flexes the elbow while applying a valgus stress to the elbow joint (Figure 3.14).

Positive Test: Pain during flexion, specifically between 30 and 60 degrees.

Indicates: Medial collateral ligament injury with or without valgus instability.

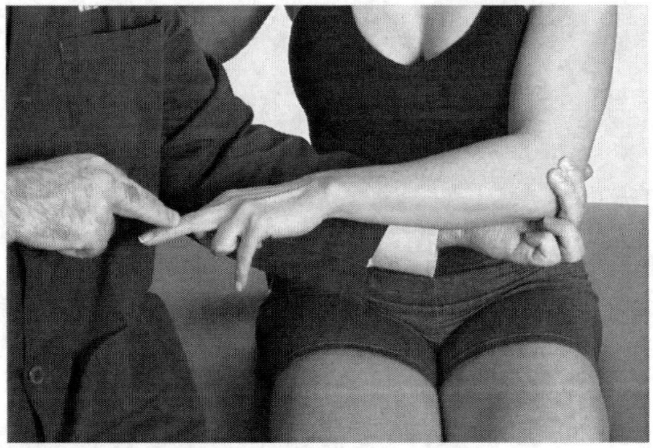

Figure 3.15. Maudsley's Test.

Maudsley's Test. The forearm and hand are placed parallel to the ground with the palm facing down. The examiner stabilizes the elbow and palpates the lateral epicondyle. The patient is asked to extend the middle finger against the examiners counterforce (Figure 3.15).

Positive Test: Pain at the lateral epicondyle.

Indicates: Lateral epicondylitis or radiocapitellar dysfunction.

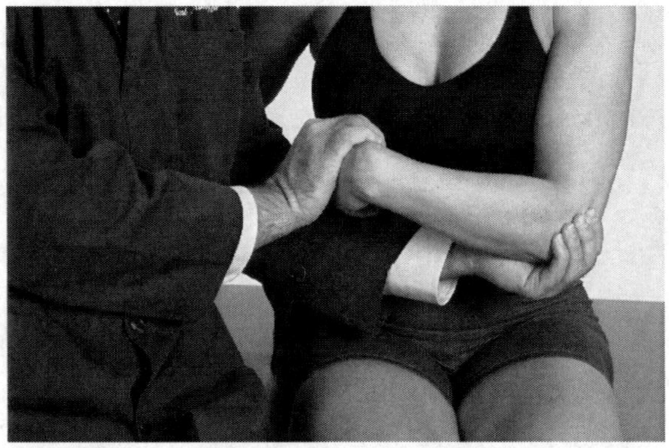

Figure 3.16. Mill's Test.

Mill's Test. The examiner flexes the patient's elbow and wrist (Figure 3.16).

Positive Test: Pain at the lateral epicondyle.

Indicates: Lateral epicondylitis or extensor muscle strain.

Posterolateral Stability

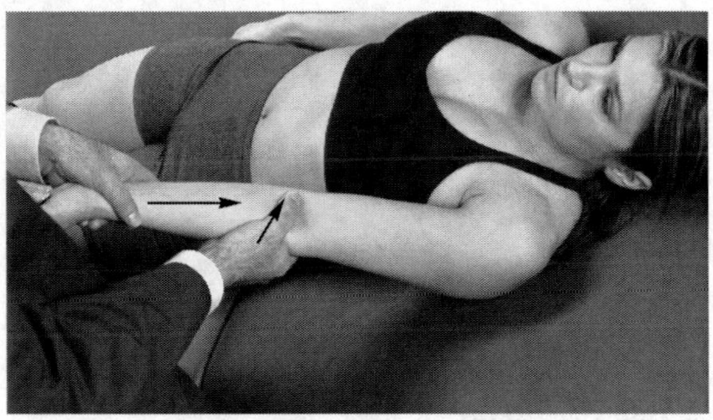

Figure 3.17. Lateral Pivot Shift Test.

Lateral Pivot Shift Test. The patient is supine with the arm slightly forward flexed and the forearm supinated. The examiner applies axial compression and valgus stress to the elbow (Figure 3.17).

Positive Test: Palpable radial subluxation, or dimpling of the skin near the radiocapitellar joint.

Indicates: Subluxation of the radial head.

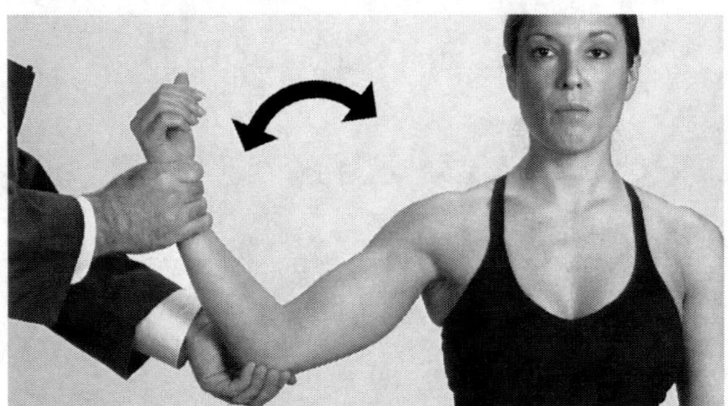

Figure 3.18. Ulnar Nerve Instability Test.

Ulnar Nerve Instability. The examiner slightly abducts and externally rotates the patient's forearm. While palpating the ulnar nerve in the ulnar groove, the examiner flexes and extends the elbow repeatedly (Figure 3.18).

Positive Test: Subluxation of the ulnar nerve in and out of its groove.

Indicates: Ulnar nerve instability.

Joint Play

Screening for radial head dysfunction can be accomplished by having the patient's elbows flexed to 90 degrees and passively pronating and supinating the forearms noting endfeel in each direction. In radial head posterior, anterior glide is restricted and the hand can pronate more easily than supinated (when compared to the opposite hand).
Conversely, in radial head anterior, posterior glide is restricted, and the hand can supinate better than pronate (when compared to the opposite hand).

COMMON CONDITIONS

- Lateral Epicondylitis (Tennis Elbow)
- Medial Epicondylitis (Golfer's Elbow)
- Olecranon Bursitis
- Valgus Extension Overload
- Cubital Tunnel Syndrome
- Panner's Disease (Osteochondrosis of the Capitellum)
- Radial Head Anterior/Posterior

Lateral Epicondylitis (Tennis Elbow)

Lateral epicondylitis is the most common overuse injury of the elbow joint. Wrist extensor muscles within the posterior compartment of the forearm share a common origin on the lateral epicondyle. Muscle tendon macroscopic tears, strain, and inflammation lead to symptoms. Specifically, the extensor carpi radialis brevis tendon is known to play a vital role in many cases. Activities involving repetitive wrist extension include the backhand serve in racquet sports as well as occupational tasks such as excessive typing. Strength imbalance between the forearm flexors and extensors may also cause lateral epicondylitis, and possibly play a role in the development of carpal tunnel syndrome. Weight lifters are often prone to this muscle imbalance because many common weight-training exercises involve the forearm flexors while neglecting the extensors.

Most patients present with pain and point tenderness over the lateral epicondyle, which may radiate down the lateral forearm. The pain is present during activities that involve the wrist extensor mechanism, such as turning a doorknob or lifting a heavy object. On examination, pain is reproducible as the patient attempts wrist or finger extension against resistance. A positive ***Maudley's Test*** and/or ***Mill's Test*** may be present.

Medial Epicondylitis (Golfer's Elbow)

Like lateral epicondylitis, this condition also results from an overuse mechanism. Several wrist and finger flexor muscles, along with the pronator teres muscle, share a common origin on the medial epicondyle. Repetitive movements involving wrist flexion or forearm pronation cause irritation surrounding the medial epicondyle. Golfers are often affected because of the nature of their swing, and by taking too many large divots placing stress on the medial elbow.

On examination, pain and tenderness is usually localized around the medial epicondyle and may radiate distally to the region overlying the pronator teres muscle. Pain is reproduced as the patient attempts to flex the wrist or fingers, or pronate the forearm against resistance.

Olecranon Bursitis

The olecranon bursa lies superficial to the posterior elbow joint. Inflammation of this fluid filled sac, termed bursitis, may be acute due to an athletic or occupational trauma or chronic due to overuse. Patients most commonly present with primary complaint of posterior elbow enlargement and distension. Often the region is painless and range of motion is normal. In cases where pain and significant decreased range of motion are detected, a septic joint must be considered.

Valgus Extension Overload

Valgus extension overload (VEO) is a condition most commonly seen in throwing athletes. A valgus stress across the elbow causes impingement of the posteromedial olecranon tip against the medial wall of the olecranon fossa. Throwers will complain of a pinpoint posteromedial elbow pain at the tip of the olecranon, which must be distinguished from MCL injury.

Cubital Tunnel Syndrome

The ulnar nerve passes behind the medial epicondyle and can be palpated in this region against the bone. Pain upon palpation may suggest ulnar irritation or neuropathy, known as cubital tunnel syndrome. There are multiple causes of cubital tunnel syndrome. Some causes include constricting fascial structures at the arcade of Struthers, subluxation of the ulnar nerve over the medial epicondyle, cubitus valgus, direct compression, spurs, tumors, and ganglia. Certain occupations have been associated with this syndrome from the repetitive motion use.

McGowan (1950) established the following classification system:

- Grade I - Mild lesions with paresthesias in the ulnar nerve distribution and a feeling of clumsiness in the affected hand; no wasting or weakness of the intrinsic muscles
- Grade II - Intermediate lesions with weak interossei and muscle wasting
- Grade III - Severe lesions with paralysis of the interossei and a marked weakness of the hand

During the physical exam, test with ***Tinel's Sign*** by tapping near the medial epicondyle in an attempt to aggravate the ulnar nerve. In addition, test with holding the elbow in maximum flexion, if symptoms of pain and numbness occur within 60 seconds of the ulnar nerve distribution this is a positive test. Froment's sign should also be performed to check the ulnar nerve function. When the patient attempts to pinch with the thumb and index finger, the flexor pollicis longus substitutes for the weak adductor pollicis. This causes the thumb to flex at the interphalangeal joint.

Panner's Disease (Osteochondrosis of the Capitellum)

Osteochondrosis is a condition resulting from alteration in the endochondral ossification centers. This condition results in interruption of blood supply to the bone, leading to avascular necrosis, and later regrowth of the bone. In the elbow, this condition may affect the medial epicondyle, olecranon, or most commonly in the capitellum of the dominant arm.

Panner's disease refers specifically to osteochondrosis of the capitellum and most commonly occurs in skeletally immature children between the ages of 4 and 12. The exact cause of Panner's disease is controversial, but overuse injuries tend to play a large role. Compressive forces placed throughout the lateral elbow joint play a role in this theory. Prognosis for this condition is very variable, and depends both on the anatomic site and on the time at which it is detected.

CONDITIONS THAT SHOULD NOT BE MISSED DUE TO MORBIDITY OR MORTALITY

- Biceps Tendon Insertion Rupture
- Triceps Tendonitis and Rupture
- Medial/Ulnar Collateral Ligament Injury
- Elbow Dislocations
- Avulsion Fracture Medial Epicondyle
- Osteochondritis Dissecans
- Supracondylar Fractures
- Forearm Fractures

Biceps Tendon Insertion Rupture

A traumatic event involving elbow flexion against resistance may result in a distal biceps tendon rupture off the radial tuberosity. Patients may reveal history of a sudden sharp pain or sensation of tearing near the anterior elbow. Examination reveals decreased flexion and supination strength, and often a swollen, painful elbow. The biceps tendon is often palpable in the antecubital fossa when a partial tear occurs, or more proximally in the arm when a complete rupture occurs.

Triceps Tendonitis and Rupture

Baseball players, weightlifters, and carpenters often perform activities requiring repetitive elbow extension. Strain is placed on the triceps tendon at its attachment to the olecranon during extension movements about the humeroulnar joint. Patients present with localized pain around the posterior elbow, and reproducible pain with resisted elbow extension.

Medial/Ulnar Collateral Ligament Injury

The medial collateral ligament, and specifically its anterior band, provides the most medial stabilization of the elbow joint. Injury to the MCL may be caused by an overuse injury or an acute valgus trauma. The MCL is a very commonly injured ligament in throwing athletes. Injury is often classified into a strain, partial tear, or full thickness tear. Clinical examination will reveal pain, and/or tenderness upon palpation and when applying a valgus stress. Increased laxity may be observed when applying valgus stress, and the degree of laxity correlates with the degree of injury. Radiographic imaging may show medial joint space widening, which is suggestive of an MCL tear.

Elbow Dislocations

Falling on an outstretched hand is the most common cause of an elbow dislocation. Posterior dislocations are much more common than anterior dislocations, and are described based on the resting position of the olecranon in relation to the humerus. The most common type of dislocation is posterolateral, followed by a pure lateral dislocation, and lastly a posteromedial dislocation.

Dislocations are further classified as either partial or complete. In a complete dislocation, it is assumed that there is complete disruption of both the medial and lateral collateral ligaments, and also the brachialis muscle is torn or significantly stretched.

Fractures may also be associated with elbow dislocations. A medial epicondyle avulsion fracture is quite common in children with open growth plates. In adults, the most commonly associated fracture is of the radial head.

Avulsion Fracture Medial Epicondyle

A valgus strain at the elbow allows traction on the medial epicondyle through the forearm flexor muscles. Severe traction may lead to an avulsion fracture of the medial epicondyle. This fracture occurs most commonly between ages 9 and 14, and is associated with elbow dislocation in half the cases.

Osteochondritis Dissecans

Osteochondritis dissecans (OCD) is an intrarticular condition of the subchondral bone, meaning it occurs within the joint and affects bone below the articular cartilage surface. Inflammation of the bone and or cartilage causes pain and may progress to cause fragmentation into the joint space.

Although the exact mechanism of injury is controversial, OCD is often associated with overuse injury or repetitive trauma, and in the elbow, is mainly localized to the capitellum of the humerus. It is commonly seen in skeletally immature adolescent males between the ages of 12 and 20 years, and specifically baseball pitchers. When throwing, the forearm is pronated during the follow-through, and excessive load is placed on the lateral elbow, specifically through the capitellum.

Patients usually complain of pain and often swelling over the lateral elbow, which is aggravated by activity and relieved by rest. With progression, decreased range of motion is noted, specifically loss of full extension. Locking and clicking may also be present, and is suggestive of osteochondral fragments, or loose bodies within the joint.

Radiographic images may show sclerotic changes in the subchondral bone around the capitellum or loose bodies within the joint. MRI or CT may also be used to confirm diagnosis. OCD lesions are described based on stability of articular cartilage and presence or lack of loose bodies.

Supracondylar Fractures

Supracondylar fractures are the most common elbow fractures among kids, and often involve an extension mechanism when falling on an outstretched hand. Fragmentation, if present, is most often displaced posteriorly.

These fractures are classified based on displacement: type I injuries are nondisplaced fractures, type II injuries are displaced fractures with cortical contact, and type III injuries are completely displaced fractures.

On examination check for associated fractures, neurological deficits of the median, radial, and ulnar nerves, peripheral pulses, and capillary refill.

Forearm Fractures

Forearm fractures in adults and children mainly result from acute trauma such as falling on an outstretched hand, and account for a majority of all childhood fractures. Any patient presenting with pain, swelling, limited range of motion, or guarding following trauma to the forearm must be evaluated for a forearm fracture.

Radiographs should include the standard anterior-posterior (AP) view and lateral view. A radiolucent triangular shadow posterior to the elbow joint on lateral radiograph is known as the posterior fat pad sign. This represents intra-articular hemorrhage and is suggestive of an occult fracture.

Radial Head Fracture - most common elbow fracture in adults

Radial Neck Fracture - more common in children than adults

Barton's Fracture - distal radius fracture with dislocation of the radiocarpal joint

Monteggia's Fracture -fracture of the proximal ulna with dislocation of the radial head

Green Stick Fracture – incomplete long bone fracture, causes the bone to bend; more common in childhood when bones are most flexible

Night Stick Fracture – ulnar shaft fracture resulting from self-defense

REFERENCES

1. Grutter P. http://www.eORIF.com. Accessed September 7, 2009.
2. Hoppenfeld S. *Physical Examination of the Spine and Extremities.* Norwalk, CT: Appleton & Lance, 1976.
3. Karageanes SJ. *Principals of Manual Sports Medicine.* Philadelphia, PA: Lippincott Wilkins & Williams; 2004.

4 The Hand and Wrist Exam

Fred H. Brennan, Jr., D.O., FAOASM

P. Gunnar Brolinson, D.O., FAOASM

Greg Beato, D.O.

Stephen Daquino, D.O., FAOASM

ANATOMY

The hand and wrist's main function is to fine tune the gross motion of the upper extremity and allow the individual to manipulate and interact with his or her environment. Additionally the hand and wrist are expressive; they serve as protection, and assist in gathering information about a person's environment through the sense of touch. Motion of the hand and wrist is accomplished through a multitude of small bones and joints, which with the assistance of multiple ligaments and both intrinsic and extrinsic muscles, allow the hand and wrist the ability to move with both precision and strength. Like any other joint in the body, freedom of movement comes at the cost of stability and vulnerability to injury. The hand and wrist are subject to many acute and chronic injuries due to this. The hand is an important instrument in any individual's activities of daily living, despite their age or activity level.

The hand and wrist are comprised of 28 bones, numerous articulations, 19 intrinsic and 20 extrinsic muscles.[1]

The palm of the hand has a few creases, which are formed by the fascial attachments of the skin to the underlying structures. They are important to know because they mark the levels of different joints of the hand. The distal palmar crease marks the MCP joints. The proximal palmar crease marks the middle of the metacarpals. The proximal interphalangeal crease indicates the PIP joints and the thenar crease defines the thenar eminence.

On the dorsal aspect of the hand the skin is attached much more loosely to allow free movement of the underlying structures. The nails should be inspected on exam of the skin. Many diseases can be reflected in the shape and condition of the nails.

The distal radioulnar joint is easily identified by following the ulna on the posteromedial side of the forearm to its termination point where it meets the expanding radius. This joint acts as a pivot to allow supination and pronation of the forearm.

Distally we find the radiocarpal joint or the wrist joint. This joint is made up of the proximal row of carpal bones where they meet the radius and ulna. The distal radius directly articulates with the scaphoid and lunate bones. The lunate and triquetrum also articulate via the triangulo fibrocartilage complex (TFCC), which originates from the ulnar radius and inserts on the ulnar styloid.[2] The TFCC provides stability to the wrist and allows part of the load from the wrist and hand to be transmitted via the ulna. Without an intact TFCC the radius would be responsible for transmission of 95% of the load placed on the wrist and hand instead of the normal 60%.[1] This joint allows for radial and ulnar deviation of the wrist as well as flexion and extension.

Stability of the carpal bones is via a complex series of ligaments. Of extreme importance amongst these ligaments is the scapholunate ligament, which is a key structure for carpal stability. This ligament is commonly injured and can lead to chronic disability if not properly diagnosed.

The intercarpal joints are located at the medial and lateral surfaces of the carpals and only allow minute sliding motions between each individual carpal bone due to the small intercarpal ligaments that bind them together. The pisiform bone sits on the palmar surface of the triquetrum and does not interact with the other carpals.[1]

The midcarpal joint is located at the junction of the proximal and distal carpal rows. They are held together by palmar and dorsal ligaments but lack the interosseous intercarpal ligaments that exist between individual bones in each row. This allows greater movement at the midcarpal joint than at the intercarpal joints. The midcarpals allow for flexion/extension as well as ulnar and radial deviation due to the formation of radial and ulnar saddle joints.

The thumb articulates with the trapezium in another sellar or saddle joint allowing 3 degrees of freedom.[1] The 2nd through 5th carpometacarpals are plane joints. The 2nd and 3rd joints are relatively immobile and confer stability to the grasp while the 4th and 5th are more mobile allowing the hand to grasp different shaped objects and allow a "power" grasp.

The intermetacarpal joints are planar joints allowing a small amount of gliding between them. The thumb does not articulate with the other metacarpals.

The metacarpalphalangeal joints are condyloid joints allowing 3 degrees of freedom at the thumb and 2 at the fingers. Ligaments on the palmar, lateral and medial sides bind the fingers. These ligaments are tightest in full flexion of the fingers.

Interphalangeal joints are uniaxial hinge joints again bound by palmar ligaments (plates) as well as medial and lateral collaterals. When fully flexed a slight bit of rotation of the fingers is induced which point each of the fingers toward the pulp of the thenar eminence. Misalignment of this relationship may indicate current or past trauma.[1]

The carpal bones of the wrist form a palmar concavity, which houses the flexors of the fingers and thumb as well as the median nerve. When capped off with the transverse carpal ligament this complex becomes known as the carpal tunnel, a common spot for nerve entrapment. Superficial to the carpal tunnel lays the tendon of the palmaris longus as well as the ulnar artey and nerve. Radially and separate from the true carpal tunnel runs the flexor carpi radialis tendon in its own compartment.

The primary movers of the wrist and hand originate from the medial and lateral epicondyles of the humerus. The tendons of the flexor digitorum profundus and superficialis traverse the carpal tunnel in close approximation to one other, the profundus runs deep to the superficialis. The extrinsic extensors of the fingers arise from the lateral epicondyle and pass under the extensor retinaculum on the dorsum of the wrist. Flexors of the hand and wrist arise from the medial epicondyle and run along the anterior forearm.

The intrinsic muscles of the hand all originate and insert within the confines of the hand (distal to the wrist crease). The intersossei muscles work together to perform adduction and abduction of the fingers. The lumbricals all run parallel to the metacarpal bones and act to assist in full extension of the PIP joints.[3]

The wrist and hand's blood supply comes from the radial, ulnar, anterior and posterior interosseous arteries.

Table 4.1. Muscles of the Hand and Wrist

	Muscle	Origin	Insertion	Action	Innervations
EXTRINSIC MUSCLES OF HAND AND WRIST	Flexor Carpi Radialis	Medial epicondyle of humerus (common flexor tendon)	Palmar Base of 2nd Metacarpal (trapezium & Base of 3rd Metacarpal)	Flex and radially deviate wrist	Median nerve
	Palmaris Longus (Inconsistent)	Medial epicondyle of humerus (common flexor tendon)	Flexor reticulaum (transverse carpal lig) and palmar aponeuosis	Wrist flexion (and thumb abduction in some people[1])	Median nerve
	Flexor Carpi Ulnaris	Humeral head-medial epicondyle of humerus (common flexor tendon) ulnar head-proximal subQ ulna	Proximal Pisiform (Flexor Retinaculum, Hamate, Base of 4th & 5th Metacarpals)	Flex and Ulnarly deviate Wrist	Ulnar nerve
	Flexor Digitorum Superficialis	3 Heads humeral head- medial Epicondyle of humerus (common flexor tendon) ulnar head- ulnar coronoid radial head- oblique line of radius	Middle phalanx of 2nd-5th digits	Flex MCP and PIP of 2nd-5th digits via split "sling" tendon, assists in flexion of wrist and elbow (each tendon is capable of independent motion)	Median nerve
	Flexor Pollicus Longus	Ventral radius, medial coronoid of ulna & adjacent interosseous memrane	Distal phalanx of thumb	Flexes the thumb	Anterior interosseous branch of median nerve

Table 4.1. Muscles of the Hand and Wrist (Continued)

	Muscle	Origin	Insertion	Action	Innervations
EXTRINSIC MUSCLES OF HAND AND WRIST	Flexor Digitorum Profundus	Medial and ventral proximal ulna, adjacent iterosseous membrane and deep fascia of forearm	Base of distal phalanxes of 2nd-4th digits	Flexes the DIP joints after the FDS flexes the PIP joints	Ulnar nerve- 4th & 5th digits anterior interosseous branch of median nerve- 2nd & 3rd digits
	Extensor Carpi Radialis Longus	Supracondylar ridge of humerus 4-5cm prox to lat epicondyle	Base of 2nd metacarpal	Extends and radially Deviates Wrist. Also assists in elbow flexion but loses some action when wrist is flexed.	Radial nerve
	Extensor Carpi Radialis Brevis	Lateral epicondyle of humerus (Common extensor tendon) and radial collateral ligament	Posterior base of 3rd betacarpal	Primary extensor of wrist. Slight radial deviation of wrist	Posterior interosseous branch of radial nerve
	Extensor Digitorum	Lateral epicondyle of humerus (Common extensor tendon)	Lateral and dorsal aspect of the 2nd-5th digits	Extends 2nd-5th digits	Posterior interosseous branch of radial nerve
	Extensor Digiti Minimi	Ulnar aspect of extensor digitorum muscle	Proximal phalanx of 5th digit	Extends 5th digit	Posterior interosseous branch of radial nerve
	Extensor Carpi Ulnaris	Lateral epicondyle of humerus (Common extensor tendon) & post border of ulna	Medial dorsal base of 5th metacarpal	Extensor of wrist in supination, ulnar deviation of wrist in pronation, works with FCU to prevent radial deviation of wrist during pronation	Posterior interosseous branch of radial nerve
	Abductor Pollicus Longus	Dorsum of proximal radius, ulna and interosseous membrane	Ventral base of 1st metacarpal	Abduction, extension and external rotation of 1st metacarpal	Posterior interosseous branch of radial nerve

Table 4.1. Muscles of the Hand and Wrist (Continued)

	Muscle	Origin	Insertion	Action	Innervations
EXTRINSIC MUSCLES OF HAND AND WRIST	Extensor Pollicus Brevis	Post radius & interosseous membrane just distal to APL	Dorsal base of proximal phalanx of thumb	Ext of prox phalanx of thumb	Posterior interosseous branch of radial nerve
	Extensor Pollicus Longus	Posterior middle ulna and interosseous membrane	Dorsal base of distal pahalanx of thumb	Ext all thumb joints; MCP, IP, CMC and helps with wrist ext	Posterior interosseous branch of radial nerve
	Extensor Indicis	Dorsum of ulna	Extensor expansion of index finger	Extension of proximal phalanx of index finger	Posterior interosseous branch of radial nerve
INTRINSIC MUSCLES OF HAND[a]	Abductor Pollicus Brevis	Flexor Retinaculum and Trapezium	Radial aspect of proximal phalanx of thumb	Abduct 1st metacarpal and prox phalanx of thumb	Median nerve
	Flexor Pollicus Brevis	Superficial head from flexor retinaculum and trapezium; deep head from floor of carpal tunnel	Base of proximal phalanx of thumb	Flexion of proximal phalanx of thumb	Superficial head from median nerve; Deep head from Ulnar nerve
	Opponens Pollicus	Flexor retinaculum and trapezium bone	Radial surface of 1st metacarpal	Flex, rotate and slightly abduct the 1st metacarpal across the palm to allow opposition	Median nerve
	Adductor Pollicus	Transverse head from ventral shaft of 3rd metacarpal; oblique head from trapezium, trapezoid and capatate and the base of 2nd and 3rd metacarpals	Ulnar side of base of proximal phalanx of the thumb	Adducts thumb and aids in opposition	Deep branch of Ulnar nerve
	Abductor Digiti Minimi	Pisiform bone and tendon of flexor carpi ulnaris	Ulnar aspect of base proximal phalanx of 5th digit	Abducts 5th digit	Deep branch of ulnar nerve
	Flexor Digiti Minimi	Flexor retinaculum and hook of hamate	Ulnar aspect of base of proximal phalanx of 5th digit	Flexion of proximal phalanx of 5th digit	Deep branch of ulnar nerve

Table 4.1. Muscles of the Hand and Wrist (Continued)

	Muscle	Origin	Insertion	Action	Innervations
INTRINSIC MUSCLES OF HAND[a]	Opponens Digiti Minimi	Flexor retinaculum and hook of hamate	Ulnar border of shaft of 5th metacarpal	Flexion and external rotation of 5th digit	Deep branch of ulnar nerve
	Palmar Interossei (3)	1st iterossei: ulnar surface of 2nd metacarpal; 2nd interossei: radial side of 4th metacarpal; 3rd interossei: radial side of 5th metacarpal	1st interossei: ulnar side of proximal phalanx of 2nd digit; 2nd interossei: radial side of proximal phalanx of 4th digit; 3rd interossei: radial side of proximal phalanx of 5th digit	Adducts the digit to which it is attached toward the middle finger and extend the distal them middle phalanges	Deep branch of ulnar nerve
	Dorsal Interossei (4)	Via 2 heads from adjacent sides of the metacarpal bones	1st interossei: radial side of proximal phalanx of 2nd digit; 2nd interossei: radial side of proximal phalanx of 3rd digit; 3rd interossei: ulnar side of proximal phalanx of 3rd digit; 4th interossei: ulnar side of proximal phalanx of 4th digit	Abduct the index, middle and ring fingers from midline of the hand	Deep branch of ulnar nerve
	Lumbricals (4- Occasionally more)	Flexor digitorum profundus tendons	Dorsal hood apparatus	IP joint extension with MCP joint in extension; assist in MCP flexion	1 & 2: median nerve; 3 & 4: ulnar nerve

a Much of Muscle chart derived from text of *Orthopaedic Examination, Evaluation and Intervention*; Dutton.[6]

The FDS and FDP tendons of the 2nd - 5th digits are held in close approximation to the phalanges by a series of 5 dense annular pulleys (A1, A2, A3, A4 & A5) and 3 thinner cruciform pulleys (C1, C2 & C3) to prevent bowstringing of the tendons.

PHYSICAL EXAM

Physical exam of the hand and wrist should begin proximally and continue distally. There is no standard order specific tests should be performed, or structures palpated, but instead the examiner should devise a systematic approach and repeat it the same way for each physical exam he or she performs. This is to ensure the examiner never misses a particular structure or test. Find a flow that works for you, and as long as it is complete, do it that way until it becomes second nature.

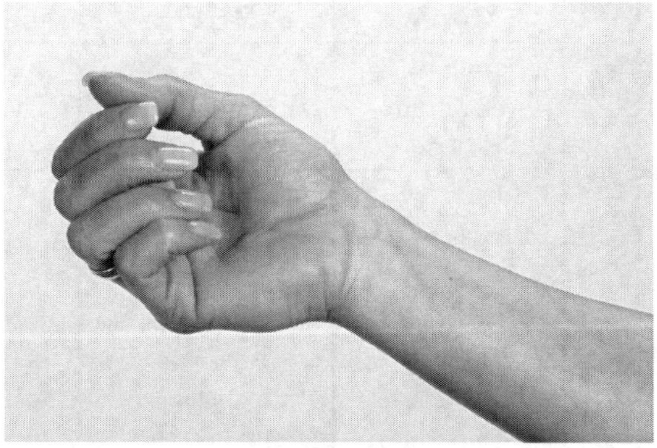

Figure 4.1. Normal attitude of the hand with fingers in flexion.

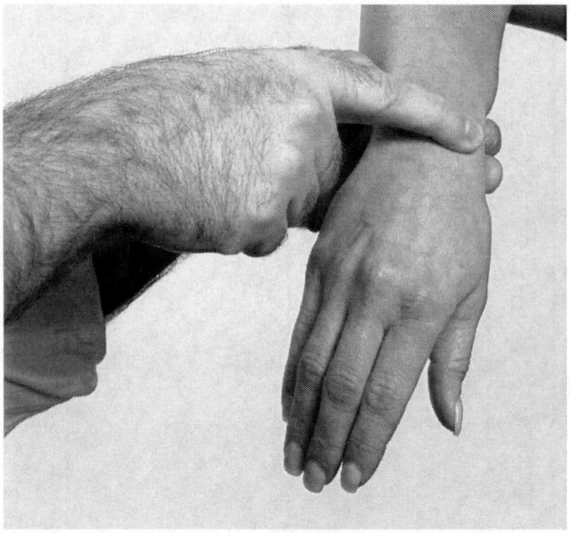

Figure 4.2. Palpation of the radial styloid.

Observation

The first component of the physical exam is gross inspection. Watch the patient enter the exam room if possible. Observe his or her gait. Does the hand and wrist swing freely with each step, or does the subject guard or protect the injured limb? Is there any gross swelling or deformity of the hand or wrist that is obvious from a distance, or subtly when compared with uninvolved hand/wrist? Sometimes the "big picture" findings may be missed if the examiner moves to a close up and detailed exam too quickly. The normal hand is carried with the fingers in a slightly flexed position (Figure 4.1). Any deviation may indicate injury. Look for any ecchymosis, swelling, or discoloration of the hand, which may indicate a recent trauma or other medical problems. A quick inspection of the nails may reveal grooves or lines due to prior trauma to the nail plates or many other findings of systemic disease.

Palpation

Each bony structure throughout the wrist and hand should be isolated and palpated. Start most distally from the injured area to prevent pain to your subject. Start with the radial (Figure 4.2) and ulnar styloids noting any swelling, deformity or pain as you palpate. Just distal to the radial styloid is the anatomic "snuffbox" (Figure 4.3). At the floor of the snuffbox lies the scaphoid bone. The scaphoid is the most frequently fractured bone in the wrist. It is a slow healing bone and notorious for delayed or non-union to occur even when identified and immobilized early after injury.

Next the wrist is guided into ulnar deviation and the proximal carpal row is palpated along the dorsal surface of the wrist. The distal carpal row should be palpated starting just distal to the scaphoid at the trapezium. The hook of the hamate can be felt prominently on the palmar suface of the wrist (Figure 4.4) and forms the ulnar border of Guyon's canal, which contains the ulnar nerve and artery.

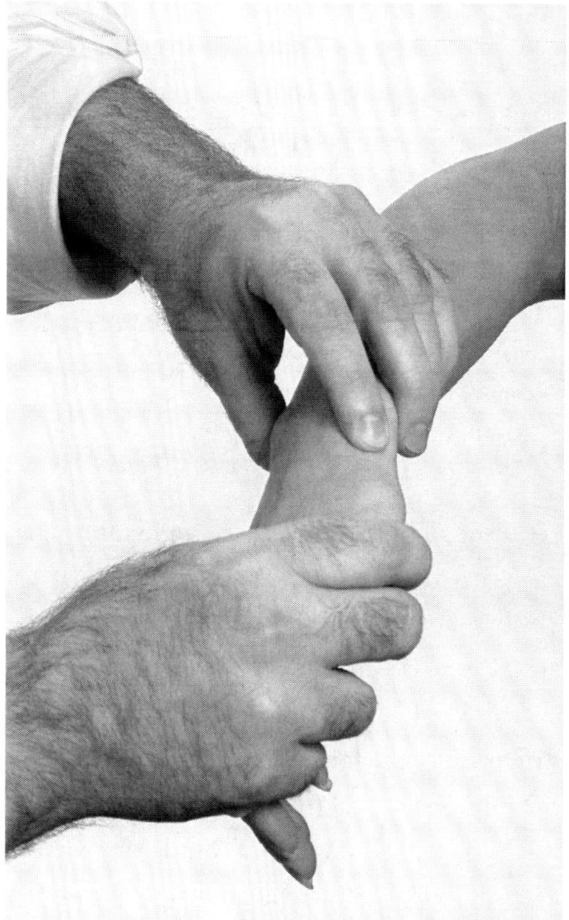

Figure 4.3. Palpation of the anatomic "snuffbox."

The bony structures and joints of the fingers and thumb should be palpated individually. Swelling, deformity, pain, warmth or crepitus should be noted.

The soft tissue structures of the hand and wrist include skin, subcutaneous fat and the major flexor/extensor tendons. These should be isolated as well as possible and palpated individually. The examiner should also palpate each of the finger pads for stability, tenderness and swelling. Intrisic muscles of the hand on the thenar and hypothenar eminences should also be palpated for swelling, tenderness and atrophy/deformity. Note any swelling, tenderness or nodularities. Soft, rubbery or fluid filled masses may indicate ganglion cysts overlying the tendon sheaths or joint lines. Hard nodules over the fingers may be indicative of arthritic conditions or gouty arthritis. Firm nodules over the flexor tendons of the fingers near the metacarpophalangeal joints may make the examiner suspicious for trigger fingers.

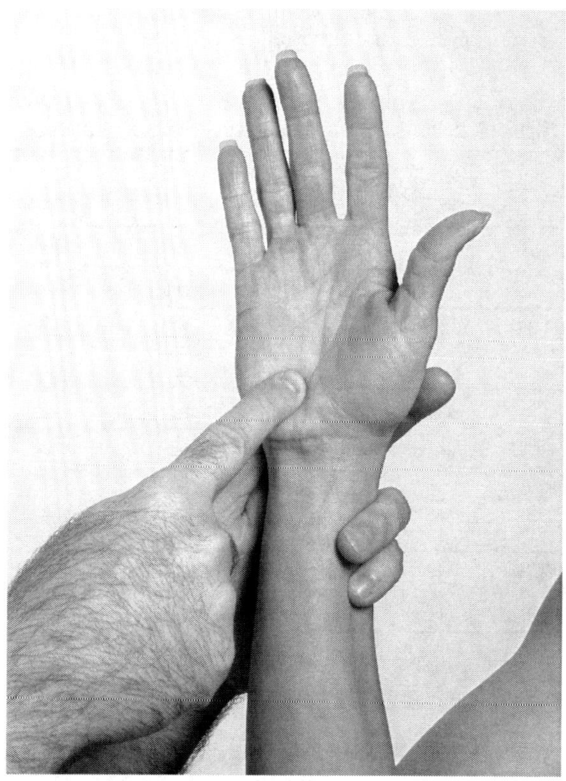

Figure 4.4. Palpation of hook of hamate.

Range of Motion

The wrist can then be moved through its range of motion. Flexion, extension, ulnar deviation, radial deviation, supination and pronation should each be tested actively and passively. Note any restrictions in range of motion and always compare to the opposite side.

Document ROMs in degrees and compare with uninvolved side.

Table 4.2. Ranges of Motion for the Wrist[a]

Motion	ROM (degrees)
Flexion	80
Extension	70
Ulnar Deviation	30
Radial Deviation	20
Supination	90
Pronation	90

[a] From Karageanes; *Principles of Manual Sports Medicine*: pg. 243.

Next the fingers should be observed through their range of motion actively, followed by passive range of motion. The range of motion of the hand is examined by having the patient make a fist and observing for any deficits. All fingers should point toward the thenar eminence and scaphoid with a normal clenched fist. Any abnormalities should be noted and further evaluated. The typical range of motion of the hand includes finger and thumb flexion and extension at the metacarpal-phalangeal joint (MCP). Finger and thumb flexion and extension at the interphalangeal (both DIP and PIP) joints, finger and thumb abduction and adduction at the MCP joints, and finger and thumb opposition. It is important when performing passive range of motion to isolate each individual joint as well as possible. This will aid in evaluating a joint's true individual ROM without the influence of the more distal and proximal joints. Without proper isolation, a joints ROM may appear greater than it actually is due to the recruitment of the joints proximal and distal to it.

Table 4.3. Active and Passive Finger Ranges of Motion[a]

Joint	Motion	Active ROM (degrees)	Passive ROM (degrees)
MCP	Flexion	95	100
	Extension	30	35
PIP	Flexion	90	100
	Extension	0	10
DIP	Flexion	90	90
	Extension	0	20
Thumb IP	Flexion	90	90
	Extension	20	20
Thumb MCP	Flexion	50	50
	Extension	10	10

[a] From Karageanes; *Principles of Manual Sports Medicine*: pg. 244.

A few small degrees of rotation, as well as adduction and abduction, are normal at each of the individual IP and MCP joints of the fingers. These small accessory motions are referred to as

"Joint Play" and can be tested individually at each joint. They are checked by the collateral ligaments on the ulnar and radial side of each joint, as well as by the volar plates on the palmar joint surface. These small accessory motions make the surface of the hand very accommodating to irregularly shaped objects, giving us much more freedom to grasp and manipulate them.

Neurovascular

Sensation is tested at the base of the thumb on the dorsal side of the hand (radial nerve), the little finger (ulnar nerve), and the index finger (median nerve). The dermatomal distribution of nerve roots can then be assessed. C6 supplies sensation to the dorsal and volar thumb and the thenar eminenece. C7 supplies the dorsal 1st web space and middle fingers from the ulnar side of the thumb to the index and middle fingers and the skin overlying their metacarpals. C7 innervates the dorsal and volar ring and little fingers as well as the ulnar aspect of the palm.[4]

Motor testing of the hand and wrist should be tested as well. Gross motor testing is accomplished with a simple grip test. Note the strength from each of the digits as the patient grasps the examiners fingers. Next individual nerves can be tested via their respective muscle innervations.

Table 4.4. Motor Testing of the Wrist and Hand[a]

Motion		Muscles		Innervation
Wrist Extension		Extensor Carpi Radialias Longus and Brevis Extensor Carpi Ulnaris		Radial Nerve
Wrist Flexion		Flexor Carpi Ulnaris		Ulnar Nerve
		Flexor Carpi Radialis (Stronger)		Median Nerve
Finger Extension		Extensor Digitorum Communis Extensor Indicis Extensor Digiti Minimi		Radial Nerve
Thumb Extension	MCP	Extensor Pollicis Brevis		Radial Nerve
	IP	Extensor Pollicis Longus		
Finger Flexion	MCP	Radial 2 Lumbricals		Median Nerve
		Ulnar 2 Lumbricals		Ulnar Nerve
	PIP	Flexor Digitorum Superficialis		Median Nerve
	DIP	Flexor Digitorum Profundus		Ulnar Nerve
Thumb Flexion	MCP	Flexor Pollicis Brevis	Medial Side	Ulnar Nerve
			Lateral Side	Median Nerve
	IP	Flexor Pollicis Longus		Median Nerve
Finger Adduction		Volar Iterossei		Ulnar Nerve
Thumb Adduction		Adductor Pollicis		Ulnar Nerve
Finger Abduction		Dorsal Interossei Abductor Digiti Minimi		Ulnar Nerve
Thumb Abduction		Abductor Pollicis Longus		Radial Nerve
		Abductor Pollicis Brevis		Median Nerve

[a] From Karageanes; *Principles of Manual Sports Medicine*: pg. 244-6.

Vascular integrity of the hand in tested by palpating the radial and ulnar pulses for strength and quality and compared with the contralateral side. The nail beds are then tested, individually if needed, for capillary refill. This is done by applying pressure to a nail bed for 4-5 seconds and then releasing it. The nail bed should blanch and then quickly return to its normal pink color as blood flows back into the capillary bed. A capillary refill time of greater than 4 seconds may indicate a compromised blood supply to the finger. Painted nails or dark pigmented individuals may alternatively have capillary refill tested at the proximal nail fold or on the finger pad if needed.

The ***Allen Test*** can be utilized to determine if there is vascular patency from both the radial and ulnar arteries to the deep and superficial palmar arches. It is accomplished by having the patient make a clenched fist, effectively squeezing the blood from the hand and then releasing the fist as the examiner occludes both the radial and ulnar arteries. The examiner then releases one of the arteries while continuing to occlude the other.

If the hand pinks up within three to five seconds then circulatory flow is considered adequate. If not, the ***Allen Test*** is positive, indicating circulatory deficit in the artery, which was just released. The test is then repeated for the other artery. The other hand can be used as a comparison when evaluating the traumatized hand.

PROVOCATIVE TESTS AND MANUEVERS

Finger Flexor Test. Flexor digitorum superficialis is tested by stabilizing the MCP joint and having the patient flex the PIP (Figure 4.5a). The flexor digitorum profundus is examined by stabilizing the PIP and having the patient flex the DIP (Figure 4.5b).

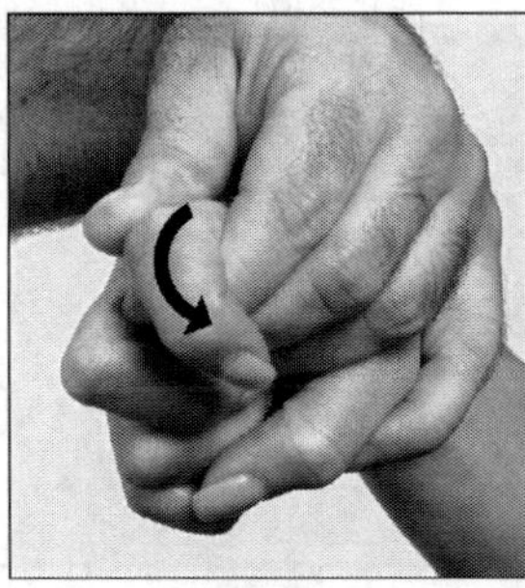

Figure 4.5a. Testing of the flexor digitorum superficialis.

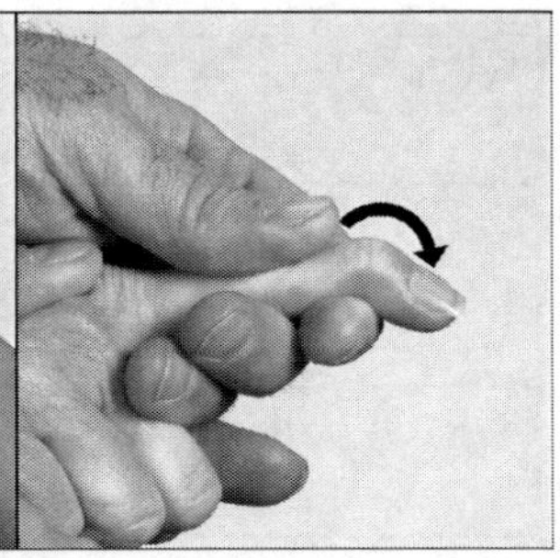

Figure 4.5b. Testing of the flexor digitorum profundus.

Positive Test: Loss of flexion at the target joint.

Indicates: FDS or FDP damage, depending on the isolated joint.

Finklestein's Test - BASIC EXAM. Utilized to assess for tenosynovitis of the 1st dorsal compartment or what is commonly referred to as DeQuervain's syndrome. The examiner asks the patient to make a fist encompassing their thumb. The examiner then ulnarly deviates the wrist (Figure 4.6).

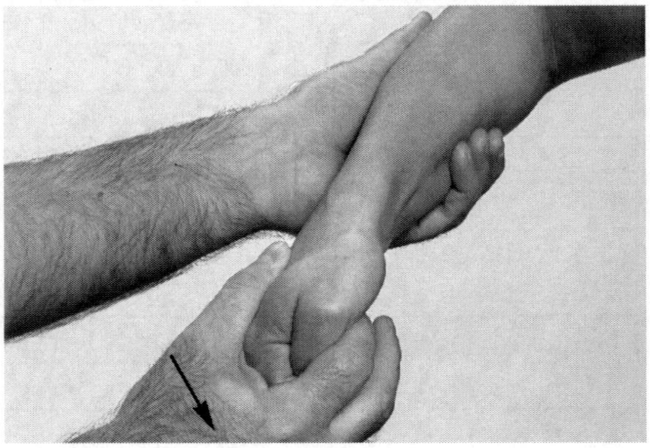

Figure 4.6. Finkelstein's Test.

Positive Test: Increased pain in the area of the first dorsal compartment.

Indicates: DeQuervain's tenosynovitis.

To physically test for median nerve entrapment (Carpal Tunnel Syndrome) a few tests can be utilized.

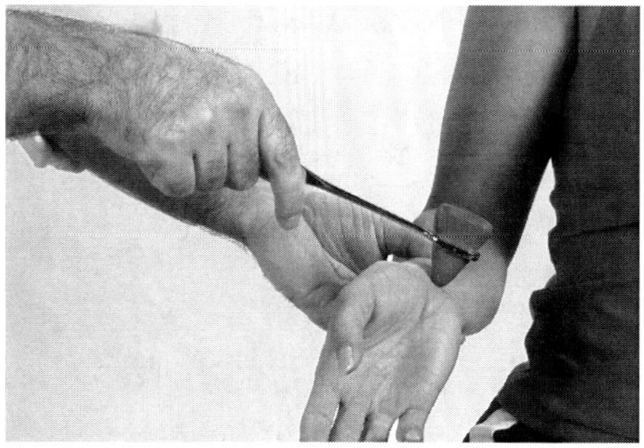

Figure 4.7. Tinel's Sign.

Tinel's Sign - BASIC EXAM. Indicates an entrapment of the Median Nerve or Carpal Tunnel Syndrome. It can be elicited by tapping over the transverse carpal ligament with either the tip of the examiners finger, or a reflex hammer, with the patient's wrist held in extension (Figure 4.7).

Positive Test: Tingling or a shock-like pain radiating to the thumb, index and middle finger and possibly up the arm.

Indicates: Carpal Tunnel Syndrome.

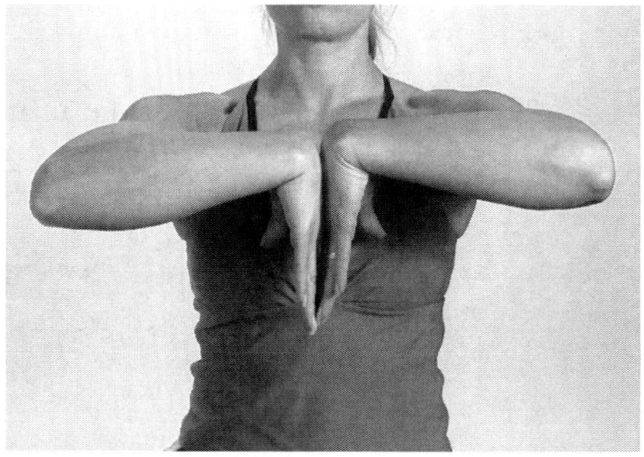

Figure 4.8. Phalen's Test.

Phalen's Test - BASIC EXAM. Accomplished by placing the dorsal aspects of the hands together and forcing them into wrist flexion (Figure 4.8). The patient holds the position for 30 to 60 seconds.

Positive Test: Any reproduction of symptoms in the distribution of the median nerve.

Indicates: Carpal Tunnel Syndrome.

Reverse Phalen's Test. This may also be utilized by having the patient place the palms together, fingers extended, and wrists dorsiflexed. This position is once again maintained for 30-60 seconds.

Positive Test: Reproduction of symptoms in the median nerve distribution.

Indicates: Carpal Tunnel Syndrome.

Carpal Compression Test. Accomplished by placing the examiner's index and middle finger pads over the transverse carpal ligament and then flexing the patient's wrist over the examiner's fingers. Again the position is held for approx 30 to 60 seconds.

Positive Test: Pain, numbness, and/or paresthesias in the median nerve distribution of the hand.

Indicates: Median nerve entrapment (Carpal Tunnel Syndrome).

Watson's Clunk Test. With the wrist in ulnar deviation, palm down, the examiner places his or her thumb over the volar aspect of the scaphoid. While maintaining pressure on the scaphoid, the wrist is passively moved into radial deviation (Figure 4.9).

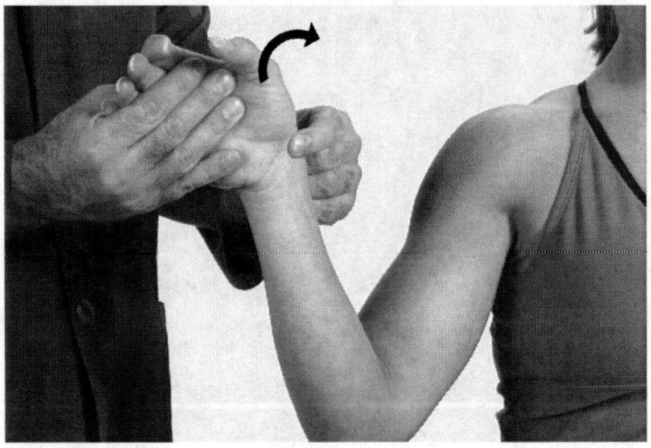

Figure 4.9. Watson's Test.

Positive Test: A painful click or clunk.

Indicates: Scapho-lunate dissociation.

Shuck Test. The patient's wrist is supported by the examiner with about 30 degrees of flexion at the wrist. The patient is asked to extend his or her fingers against the examiner's resistance.

Positive Test: Pain over the area of the lunate.

Indicates: Peri-lunate instability.

Evaluation of the Ulnar Collateral Ligament - BASIC EXAM. With the MP joint of the thumb isolated, the examiner attempts to abduct the joint.

Positive Test: Laxity or pain over the ulnar side of the MP joint.

Indicates: Sprain of the Ulnar Collateral Ligament of the thumb (Gamekeeper's or Skiier's Thumb).

Evaluation of Triangular Fibrocartilage Complex - BASIC EXAM.

COMMON CONDITIONS

- Mallet Finger
- Metacarpal Fracture
- PIP Dislocation
- Distal Radius Fracture
- Distal Ulna Fracture
- Carpal Tunnel Syndrome
- DeQuervain's Tenosynovitis
- Trigger Finger
- Ulnar Collateral Ligament tears of thumb (Gamekeeper's or Skier's Thumb)
- TFCC Tears
- Ganglion Cysts
- Phalanx Fractures

Mallet Finger

Typically referred to as a "jammed finger," a mallet finger is a disruption of the distal extensor tendon and ligament that occurs when an object forcefully contacts the tip of the finger. This usually is moderately painful immediately and will become swollen and bruised. On examination the patient will be unable to actively fully straighten the distal interphalangeal (DIP) joint, making it look flexed (hence the term "mallet finger"). All the other interphalangeal joints should be thoroughly evaluated to make certain other damage is not present. Radiographic evaluation should be performed to determine if there is an avulsion fracture ("bony mallet"). There are several different classification schemes, largely based on size of fragment and involvement of the articular surface.

Teaching Point: The typical jammed finger may result in an extensor tendon disruption and/or an avulsion fracture. If the tip of the digit cannot be extended, and/or droops, a mallet finger injury should be suspected. This will require prolonged splinting and therefore should be recognized.

Metacarpal Fracture

The most common metacarpal fracture is known as a "boxer's fracture," and involves the fifth metacarpal. This can occur from an incorrectly thrown punch, resulting in a fracture to the distal metacarpal neck. There are multiple other potential mechanisms of injury described in the literature as well. Due to traction from the interosseous muscles, the proximal and smaller fragment usually displaces in the volar direction.

Physical examination will reveal tenderness, edema, ecchymosis, and possibly a deformity at the more distal end of the metacarpal. One must assess for rotation of the affected metacarpal by having the patient make a fist, as best as possible, and draw an imaginary line down the distal phalanges through the tips of the fingers. These imaginary lines should all converge and intersect at the volar aspect of the scaphoid bone. Radiographic evaluation should include at least three views of the hand to assess for any angulation, displacement, and/or rotation.

Teaching Point: Always assess metacarpal fractures for any degree of angulation and/or digital rotation. Angular and rotational deformities should be evaluated by an orthopedic specialist.

Proximal Interphalangeal Joint Dislocation

Finger dislocations are common in athletics, with the proximal interphalangeal articulation being the most commonly affected joint. Usually the dislocation occurs in the dorsal direction, but it can also displace laterally or in the volar direction. Several associated injuries can occur due to the displacement, including avulsion fractures, volar plate disruptions, and tendon ruptures, depending on the direction of the dislocation. Efficient and effective treatment of these injuries can protect against improper healing and deformity.

On physical examination, the patient will be tender around the PIP joint, have swelling, and the deformity is usually obvious. After careful evaluation, the physician can attempt to reduce the dislocation on the sideline or in the training room prior to obtaining radiographs. Assuming the reduction was uncomplicated and the athlete's pain is manageable, the finger can be splinted and "buddy-taped" and the athlete may be allowed to continue in the athletic event. If the dislocation is unable to be reduced easily, or there is evidence of a fracture or neurovascular compromise, disqualification from the event is warranted so that urgent radiographs and orthopedic or hand surgeon evaluation can be obtained. After reduction, radiographs should be obtained to ensure proper alignment and assess for occult fracture. One must test the integrity of the flexor and extensor tendons, and collateral ligaments, post-reduction.

Teaching Point: Athletes who sustain an uncomplicated, non-fracture PIP joint dislocation may be allowed to return to activity post successful reduction if the joint can be protected and the pain is tolerable.

Distal Radius Fracture

The radius is the most commonly fractured arm bone and occurs most often as a result of a fall on the outstretched hand (FOOSH). Other potential mechanisms include direct trauma, motor vehicle collisions, and skiing and bike accidents. Occasionally the ulna is also fractured concurrently with the radial fracture. There are several different types of distal radius fractures, depending on the direction of the fracture (dorsal or volar), involvement of the articular surface (intra-articular or extra-articular), associated carpal bone and soft tissue injury, angulation, comminution, and involvement of the ulna. Also, there are several different classification systems, including the Frykman, Melone, and Universal classifications. Each of these emphasizes different aspects of the fracture and its potential implication for treatment and recovery.

Typically the patient will present with moderate to severe pain and swelling in the wrist, often times with an obvious deformity. The wrist will be splinted and supported by the unaffected hand and likely braced against the body for comfort and to limit motion. On exam, wrist range of motion will be significantly limited by pain and potentially the displaced fracture fragment. One must be thorough in inspecting for any skin breakages, as this may indicate an open fracture, which has more urgent treatment implications. After inspection and palpation, noting the specific areas of deformity and tenderness, and a careful assessment of the active and then passive ranges of motion, one must perform a thorough neurovascular examination. Attention to the median nerve, including its branch the anterior interosseous nerve, and the posterior interosseous branch, off the radial nerve, is essential in the physical examination. Vascular examination includes direct palpation of the radial and ulnar artery, comparing strength of pulsation to the contralateral side, capillary refill, and the Allen's test.

Teaching Point: A complete evaluation and assessment of the forearm and elbow should also be performed to evaluate for other injuries, including further fractures, dislocations, or compartment syndrome.

Distal Ulnar Fracture

A fracture to the distal ulna is called a nightstick fracture because of the reflex to protect one's head with the forearm when attacked with a night stick or other object. Many of these fractures are "stable" (less than 50% displaced) because of the many soft tissue attachments, like the periosteum, interosseous membrane, and muscular attachments. If evaluating and treating "unstable" (more that 50% displaced or 10-15 degrees of angulation) fractures one must also assess for a proximal radial head dislocation (Monteggia fracture) and/or fracture.

Physical examination includes gentle palpation for the deformity, as the patient will most likely be in significant pain and will protect/guard the area. Inspect the area for edema, ecchymosis, and skin surface disruption. Motion testing will likely be limited, especially pronation and supination of the wrist. Always assess distal pulses, capillary refill, and perform a thorough neuro-sensory exam.

Teaching Point: Distal forearm fractures are usually not subtle and likely very painful. Without displacement or other complications these can be treated with immobilization for 4-6 weeks, with periodic imaging to document healing.

Carpal Tunnel Syndrome

Entrapment of the median nerve at the wrist, in the carpal tunnel, produces pain, numbness, tingling, reduced motion, and possibly atrophy of the intrinsic muscles of the hand. This is known as carpal tunnel syndrome. Some of the most common identified causes of Carpal Tunnel Syndrome are pregnancy, metabolic disorders like diabetes mellitus and hypothyroidism, trauma, and osteoarthritis. Overuse is another common etiology and the most typical predisposing factor for sports related carpal tunnel syndrome. The typical presentation early on in the disorder is numbness and tingling in the thumb, index, and middle fingers. Symptoms classically are worse at night. Often times the patient will complain of decreased grip strength and a sensation of fullness in the hand and wrist. In more chronic cases patients notice atrophy of the thenar musculature.

Classically, the physical examination of a patient with Carpal Tunnel Syndrome will produce neuropathic symptoms with direct tapping on the carpal tunnel (Tinel's Test). Phalen's test is another common diagnostic maneuver where both wrists are maximally palmar flexed at the same time by pressing together the dorsal aspects of the hands (reverse prayer position), and holding for 30 to 60 seconds. Progressive numbness and/or tingling in this position is a positive test. Examination should also include forearm and wrist range of motion and motor strength, along with complete sensory evaluation. The gold standard in diagnosing carpal tunnel syndrome is electromyography and nerve conduction velocity. This study will demonstrate slowed conduction of the median nerve at the carpal tunnel and in the hand. However, carpal tunnel syndrome is most often diagnosed by clinical history and examination.

Teaching Point: Carpal Tunnel Syndrome is common. Physicians should always consider potential underlying disease states and treat those conditions as well. Carpal Tunnel Syndrome will often resolve with conservative measures to include OMT, bracing, and occupational therapy.

DeQuervain's Tenosynovitis

Pain and inflammation from repetitive overuse of tendons in the first dorsal compartment of the wrist is DeQuervain's tenosynovitis. The first dorsal compartment of the wrist has a tendon sheath that encompasses the abductor pollicis longus and the extensor pollicis brevis tendons at the lateral border of the anatomical snuffbox. Although occasionally injured with an isolated acute traumatic event, this area is most commonly injured as a result of repetitive movements involving the wrist and thumb. Patients will often complain of dorsal-lateral wrist and thumb pain, occasionally with radiation into the lateral hand and thumb. A carful history about repetitive activities, including vocational and recreational, is essential.

Physical examination of the patient with dorsal-lateral wrist and thumb pain includes palpation of the affected and surrounding areas, especially the snuffbox, complete hand and wrist muscle testing, neuro-vascular evaluation, and special tests. Classically, the Finkelstein test is the physical examination maneuver that will recreate pain of DeQuervain's tenosynovitis. This test is performed by having the patient make a fist around the tucked thumb, and then passively ulnarly deviating the wrist. This maneuver will create pain over the first dorsal compartment of the wrist; a positive test.

Teaching Point: Tenderness over the tendons that approximate the radial styloid process of the wrist is often due to Dequervain's tenosynovitis.

Trigger Finger

A triggering finger, or trigger finger, occurs when a digital flexor tendon becomes restricted in motion due to inflammation and/or scarring of the tendon or its sheath. Trigger finger is usually caused by repetitive grasping of the fingers. It occurs with repetitive painting or racquet sports, or in patients with autoimmune or inflammatory conditions, diabetes mellitus, or rheumatoid arthritis. The digit may become "stuck" in a flexed position. Often times the flexed tendon will pop as it snaps, or "triggers," under the A-1 pulley. The A-1 pulleys are located over the palmar aspects of the metacarpal-phalangeal joints. All fingers should be examined, as well as a complete neurovascular evaluation of the hands.

Teaching Point: Although treating the underlying pathology is important, trigger fingers respond well to local corticosteroid injections. In some recalcitrant cases, surgical debridement may be necessary.

CONDITIONS THAT SHOULD NOT BE MISSED DUE TO POSSIBLE MORBIDITY OR MORTALITY

- Scaphoid Fracture
- Scapho-Lunate Dissociation
- Jersey Finger (Flexor Tendon Disruption)
- Hook of the Hamate Fracture
- PIP Extensor Central Slip Tear/Boutonnière Deformity
- Compartment Syndrome of Hand
- Open Fractures of the Hand/Wrist

Scaphoid Fracture

Scaphoid or carpal navicular fractures are common in athletics and represent the most common carpal bone fracture. The mechanism of injury is typically from falling forward or backwards on an outstretched hand. Fractures of the scaphoid bone can be challenging to diagnose. Initial x-rays can be deceivingly negative. Having a high index of suspicion, based on an accurate history and physical, is crucial. A delay in diagnosis and proper treatment can predispose the patient to a delayed or non-union, osteoarthritis of the radiocarpal joint, and decreased function of the wrist due to pain and loss of motion.

The patient will often complain of a dull achiness deep in the radial aspect of the wrist after sustaining a fall. Examination will reveal decreased wrist range of motion, decreased grip strength, and tenderness in the "anatomical snuff box" that overlies the scaphoid bone. Fullness in the snuff box may be appreciated due to joint swelling. Tenderness may also be elicited by palpating in the snuffbox while dorsiflexing the wrist, as well as resisting pronation and ulnar deviation. Axial compression or loading through the thumb into the scaphoid bone may also produce pain.

Patients sustaining a fall on an outstretched hand, with tenderness around the anatomical snuffbox, should always have radiographs to exclude potential fracture. An anterior-posterior (AP), true lateral, and scaphoid view are the minimum views to obtain. An obvious scaphoid fracture may not be present on the initial radiographs.

Teaching Point: A fall on an outstretched hand with resultant anatomical snuffbox tenderness is a scaphoid fracture until proven otherwise. A negative x-ray does not rule out the diagnosis. Immobilize the wrist with a thumb spica cast/splint and re-examine in two weeks. Persistent pain requires referral.

Scapho-Lunate Dissociation

As the most common cause of carpal joint instability, a scapho-lunate dissociation can cause significant pain and limitation due to disruption of the scapho-lunate ligament and soft tissue connections. The injury mechanism is similar to that causing a scaphoid fracture, a fall on an outstretched hand. There is a spectrum of severity included in this injury, ranging from dynamic instability to scapho-lunate advanced collapse. The term scapho-lunate dissociation is used when a scapho-lunate ligament tear leads to a rotational dislocation of the scaphoid from the adjacent lunate. Dorsal wrist pain and limitation of dorsi and palmar flexion are common presenting symptoms…similar to a scaphoid fracture. A delay in diagnosis is common as patients often treat this as a simple wrist sprain.

The physical examination will demonstrate dorsi-radial sided wrist pain and some degree of swelling. Range of motion, especially extension and radial deviation, may be reduced because of pain. Hand grip and resisted wrist extension strength is often limited by pain. X-rays to include an AP view, an AP with clenched fist view (accentuates potential instability/separation between the scaphoid and lunate bones), a true lateral, and a scaphoid view are essential. A separation of 3 millimeters or more between the scaphoid and lunate bones on any AP view of the wrist is highly suspicion for a scapho-lunate dissociation. MRI is necessary if x-rays are inconclusive.

Teaching Point: A fall on an outstretched hand may cause a disruption of the scapho-lunate ligament. If tenderness over the scapho-lunate region of the dorsal wrist is noted then x-rays, including an AP clenched fist view and true lateral view, should be taken. A three-millimeter space between the scaphoid and lunate bone and/or an asymmetry of the two wrists on x-rays is suspicious for scapho-lunate dissociation.

Jersey Finger or Flexor Tendon Rupture

A disruption of the flexor digitorum profundus (FDP) tendon near the distal interphalangeal (DIP) joint results in an inability to actively flex the distal phalanx. Jersey finger, as the nickname implies, typically occurs when an athlete attempts to make a tackle and gets his/her finger caught in the opponent's jersey. The FDP may stretch, completely rupture, or avulse a bony fragment from the distal phalanx. The patient will complain of pain and swelling at or near the DIP joint. The physical examination will reveal tenderness, edema and a possible deformity on the volar aspect of the DIP. The proximal interphalangeal joint (PIP) of the injured finger should be held in a neutral position as the patient attempts to flex only the DIP joint. The patient will not be able to flex the DIP joint or will have demonstrable weakness with attempts at flexing the fingertip. Radiographic evaluation should include AP, lateral, and oblique views of the affected finger to assess for fractures.

Teaching Point: Pain, weakness, and/or an inability to flex the tip of the finger after a hand injury should make the clinician suspicious for a jersey finger (FDP), injury.

Splinting and prompt consultation should be obtained for a suspected a jersey finger injury.

Hook of the Hamate Fracture

The hamate bone of the wrist is unique having a small hook that can be palpated on the palmar-ulnar side of the hand. Because of its location, it is somewhat vulnerable to injury. Trauma to the hamate may occur from a direct fall on an outstretched hand, swinging a baseball bat, or from swinging a golf club making unexpected contact with the hard ground. The patient typically experiences acute pain over the hamate and may even experience an appreciable "pop" if the hook fractures.

The physical exam typically reveals direct tenderness and swelling over the ulnar-palmar aspect of the hand near the distal palmar crease. Palmar flexion and ulnar deviation tends to exacerbate the pain. Direct pressure and/or attempts to swing a baseball bat or golf club produces ulnar wrist pain. An anterior-posterior (AP), lateral, and carpal tunnel radiographic views of the wrist will demonstrate the fracture of the hook of the hamate and rule out other carpal bone injury.

Teaching Point: Ulnar-palmar wrist pain due to a fall, swinging a baseball bat, or swinging a golf club should raise suspicion of an injury to the hook of the hamate. Wrist x-rays to include a carpal tunnel view should be done to exclude an occult fracture.

PIP (Proximal Interphalangeal) Extensor Central Slip Tear/Boutonnière Deformity

Patients often report having their fingers "jammed" by either a fall or an object hitting their extending fingers. For example, a basketball player may jam their finger trying to catch a passed ball. The patient reports pain over the dorsum of the PIP joint of the injured digit. The joint is often swollen, red, and has limited motion due to the pain and swelling. This injury is often treated simply with ice, analgesics, and buddy taping the injured finger to an adjacent finger. However, overlying the joint is a central extensor slip aiding in PIP joint extension. That central slip may be torn when the finger is jammed and must be assessed to prevent long-term disability.

The physical exam of the jammed digit must include palpation of the bony structures, ligament stability testing, and testing the integrity of the flexor and extensor mechanisms. X-rays of the injured digit should be performed to rule out bony fracture or avulsion. Injury to the extensor central slip may be detected by resisting the finger as the patient gently attempts to extend it. If there is demonstrable weakness in extension strength or significant pain over the dorsum of the joint then a central slip injury should be suspected.

Teaching Point: A "jammed" finger may be more than just a simple joint sprain. After negative radiographs always assess the extensor mechanism of that injured joint; both strength and pain. If there is demonstrable weakness and/or more than expected discomfort, splint the joint in extension and refer for further evaluation.

Compartment Syndrome of Hand

Significant trauma to the hand resulting in multiple bone fractures and/or soft tissue damage may result in compartment syndrome of the hand. Trauma of this magnitude may lead to large amount of swelling in the hand. Swelling in the compartment leads to increases in compartmental pressures. Subsequently neurovascular compromise ensues. A patient may first complain of worsening pain, decreasing sensation, or a feeling of "pins and needles." The hand may feel tight and any passive stretching or movement of the flexor/extensor tendons intensifies the pain. If untreated, the hand will become pulseless, ischemic, and potentially non-viable.

Teaching Point: Any crush injury, paint gun injury, or injury involving multiple fractures of the hand should be monitored closely for evolving signs and symptoms of compartment syndrome. Worsening pain, numbness, pain out of proportion to the injury, and pain with passive tendon stretch is an evolving compartment pressure until proven otherwise. Urgent surgical consultation is critical.

Open Fractures of the Hand/Wrist

An open fracture, once named a compound fracture, is a fracture that has compromised the integrity of the skin. Sometimes these fractures are obvious as the skin is clearly disrupted. However sometimes only a small split in the skin surface is observed, or a finger tip/nail is crushed. If the fingernail is split and the underlying bone is fractured (distal phalynx) then an open fracture must be assumed. If a fracture is seen on an x-ray, look closely at the overlying soft tissue shadows to see if there is tissue compromise communicating with the fracture site. Open fractures should be carefully explored for gross contamination and thoroughly irrigated...often in the operating room. A contaminated open fracture places the soft tissue and underlying bone at risk for developing an infection. Osteomyelitis (bone infection) and deep soft tissue infections of the hand are difficult to treat with potential long-term functional impairment due to scarring and contactures.

Teaching Point: Look carefully at the hand and wrist for any signs of disruption in skin integrity at or near a fracture site. This may be a sign of an open fracture. Crush injuries to the nail/nailbed with fracture and split in the fingernail should raise high suspicion for an open fracture.

REFERENCES

1. Magee DJ. *Orthopedic Physical Assessment.* Fourth Ed. Philadelphia, PA: W. B. Saunders Company; 2002:355-8.
2. Karageanes SJ. *Principles of Manual Sports Medicine.* Philadelphia, PA: Lippincott Williams & Wilkins; 2005:232.
3. Karageanes SJ. *Principles of Manual Sports Medicine.* Philadelphia, PA: Lippincott Williams & Wilkins; 2005:238.
4. Karageanes SJ. *Principles of Manual Sports Medicine.* Philadelphia, PA: Lippincott Williams & Wilkins; 2005:244.
5. Seidenberg PH, Beutler AI. *The Sports Medicine Resource Manual.* Philadelphia, PA: Saunders Elsevier; 2008:178-215.
6. Dutton M. *Orthopaedic Examination, Evaluation & Intervention.* New York:The McGraw-Hill Companies; 2004:593.

5 The Thoracic Spine Exam

William M. Falls, Ph.D.

Gail A. Shafer-Crane, Ph.D.

Robert N. Pedowitz, D.O.

Michael Wieting, D.O.

ANATOMY

The thoracic spine, which consists of the 12 thoracic vertebrae, contains the thoracic and upper lumbar portions of the spinal cord and associated nerve roots whose branches supply the back and the anterolateral thoracic and abdominal walls in a segmental fashion from the neck to the pelvis. This region of the vertebral column serves as an attachment for the ribs and transmits the weight of the body to the lumbosacral spine. The thoracic spine is presented in detail in major anatomic textbooks.

The distinguishing feature of all 12 thoracic vertebrae is that they articulate with at least one pair of ribs. Typical thoracic vertebrae articulate with two pairs of ribs; the head of the rib contacts a facet on the superior margin of one vertebral body above. In addition, there is a facet on the transverse processes of thoracic vertebrae.

Bodies of thoracic vertebrae increase in size from T1 to T12 and display highly convex anterior surfaces, which protrude deeply into the thoracic cavity. The protrusion is exaggerated by the direction of the transverse processes, which project posteriorly and superiorly as well as laterally. The pedicles attach to the superior ends of the vertebral bodies thereby creating deep inferior vertebral notches, which accommodate the spinal nerve roots. The laminae are broad and those of the superior vertebra overlap those of the vertebra lying immediately inferior.

The long and slender spinous processes point inferiorly and overlap the vertebra lying inferiorly. The spinous processes of the lower thoracic vertebrae resemble those of lumbar vertebrae; they are shorter, stouter, and project more posteriorly. The superior and inferior articular processes are situated anterior to the transverse process and their facets are oriented in the coronal plane. The superior facet faces posteriorly and laterally, while the inferior facet faces anteriorly and medially. There is an abrupt transition in the orientation of the articular processes at the level of T12 where the inferior articular process becomes oriented to match those of the lumbar vertebrae with an anterolaterally directed facet.

There are 12 pairs of ribs, which articulate with the thoracic vertebrae through their heads and short necks. The head of a typical rib has a superior and inferior facet divided by a crest for articulation with the bodies of two adjacent thoracic vertebrae. The superior border of the narrower neck also displays a crest for the attachment of ligaments. The neck terminates laterally in an articulation tubercle, which bears an oval, convex facet for articulation with the transverse process of the similarly numbered thoracic vertebrae. Lateral to the facet is a rough area for attachment of a ligament. The tubercle marks the junction of the neck and the body of the ribs, which turns sharply forward at the angle and slants inferiorly and forward. The head of the first rib is different from the others in that it only has a single facet for articulation with the facet on the superior margin of the body of the T1 vertebra.

The thoracic spine is composed of two types of joints, which work together to provide mobility for the spine. These include facet joints (zygapohyseal joints) and intervertebral body joints (intervertebral discs). The facet joints are synovial joints between the articular processes of adjacent vertebrae. A thin, loose articular capsule surrounds each joint. The facet joints permit gliding movement between the vertebrae, and the shape of the articular surfaces limits the range of motion possible. Branches arising from the posterior primary rami of spinal nerves innervate these joints.

The intervertebral discs are fibrocartilaginois joints, designed for weight bearing and strength, situated between the bodies of adjacent vertebrae. Each intervertebral disc consists of an outer annulus fibrocartilage, which surrounds a gelatinous nucleus pulposus. The annuli insert into the rounded rims on the articular surfaces of adjacent vertebral bodies. Branches arising from the anterior primary rami of spinal nerves innervate the intervertebral disc. The intervertebral disc avascular structures receive their blood supply by diffusion from the vertebral bodies. Mobility of the thoracic spine, especially in its superior and middle regions is limited mainly due to the ribs and rib cage as well as the narrowness of the intervertebral discs. Rotation takes place primarily in the thoracic spine, with flexion, extension, and lateral bending being extremely limited.

Ligaments reinforce and stabilize the facet joints and the intervertebral discs. The anterior longitudinal ligament is a broad, thick band attaching to anterior and anterolateral surfaces of the vertebral bodies and vertebral discs. It limits extension of the vertebral column. The posterior longitudinal ligament runs within the vertebral canal and attaches to the posterior surfaces of the vertebral bodies and the intervertebral disc. In the thoracic region it narrows over the surfaces of the vertebral bodies and expands over the intervertebral disc. The posterior longitudinal ligament checks flexion of the vertebral column. The strong, highly elastic, flattened ligamenta flava attach to the laminae of adjacent vertebrae. These ligaments help to preserve the normal curvature of the vertebral column and straighten the vertebral column after it has been flexed. Short interspinous ligaments and a strong cord like supraspinous ligament joint adjacent spinous processes. The intertransverse ligaments connect adjacent transverse processes and are insignificant in the thoracic spine.

The ribs articulate with the thoracic spine at two synovial joints; the costovertebral and costotransverse joints. At the costovertebral joint, the head of a rib articulates with two vertebral bodies. A ligament attaching the crest of the head to the intervertebral disc divides the joint cavity. The articular capsules are thickened anteriorly by the radiate ligament, which anchors the head of the rib to the intervertebral disc and to the thoracic vertebral bodies superior and inferior to the disc. The costotransverse joint is between the articulating tubercle on the rib and the transverse process of the vertebra. The joint has a small cavity and is strengthened by three costotranverse ligaments. These extend between the crest on the rib neck and the transverse process superior to the rib (superior costotransverse ligament), between the posterior aspect of the rib neck and its own transverse process (costotransverse ligament), and between the tip of the transverse process and the rough part of the articulating tubercle (lateral costotransverse ligament). These joints are responsible for the pump-handle and bucket-handle movements of the ribs. Both joints receive their arterial supply from branches of the posterior intercostal arteries and are innervated by branches of the posterior primary rami of the thoracic spinal nerves.

The control and strength of movements in the thoracic spine, as well as in other regions of the spine, are dependent on muscles. Muscles help to stabilize the spine and control the effects of gravity. The extensor muscles are the one major functional group of the thoracic spine. The group is also capable of rotating and side bending the spine. Flexor muscles located on the anterior aspect of the spine in other regions are absent in the thoracic spine. The extensor muscles (deep back muscle) span the entire back from the skull to the sacrum and in the thoracic region are situated posterior to the laminae and transverse processes between the spinous processes medially and the angle of the ribs laterally. They are innervated segmentally by the posterior primary rami of the thoracic spinal nerves. These muscles consist of two groups: erector spinae and transversospinalis. The muscles are enclosed in the thin thoracic portion of the thoracolumbar fascia, which attaches to the spinous processes of the thoracic vertebrae and the angles of the ribs and separates the muscles from overlying superficial muscles. The erector spinae muscles are responsible for restoring the spine to the erect posture after flexion and also act to control flexion of the spine against gravity. The transversospinalis muscle act primarily to rotate the spine.

The erector spinae and transversospinalis muscles are arranged in three layers: superficial, intermediate and deep. In the thoracic spine, the superficial layer consists of three vertically running columns of muscles. The most lateral column is the iliocostalis, which runs along the angles of the ribs. Portions of all three subdivisions of the iliocostalis—lumborum, thoracics, and cervicis—can be found in the thoracic spine. The intermediate column is the longissimus, which is associated with the transverse processes. In the thoracic spine, the thoracis and part of the cervicis subdivisions of the thoracis muscle can be found. The medial column is the spinalis, which is associated with spinous processes. The intermediate layer is composed of two subgroups of the transversospinalis muscles. As the name of the muscle group implies, the transversospinalis muscles arise from transverse processes and insert into spinous processes.

In the thoracic spine, the intermediate layer is composed of the thoracis and cervicis portions of the semispinalis muscle and deep to them, the multifidus muscles. The semispinalis muscle span up to six vertebrae, while the multifidus muscle span two to four vertebrae. The deep layer is composed of segmental muscles: interspinous, intertransverse, and rotator groups. All of these groups are better developed in the cervical and lumbar spine than they are in the thoracic spine. The rotators typically span one to two vertebrae. In the thoracic spine the deep back muscles and the overlying thoracolumbar fascia are covered by other muscles, which are not innervated by the posterior primary rami of the thoracic spinal nerves and which attach the upper limb to the vertebral column. These include the trapezius, latissimus dorsi, and deep to the trapezius, the rhomboids.

Blood supply to the thoracic spine, associated muscles, nerve roots, and spinal cord is derived from 12 pairs of posterior intercostal arteries arising from the costocervial trunk of the subclavian artery (posterior intercostals 1 and 2) and the thoracic aorta (posterior intercostals 3 to 12), which enter and course in the intercostal spaces on the anterolateral thoracic wall. Near its origin each posterior intercostal artery gives off a posterior branch that passes posteriorly with the posterior primary rami of the corresponding thoracic spinal nerve. This branch supplies the back muscles and overlying skin as well as the thoracic spine and contributes to supply the nerve roots, the spinal cord and it coverings, and the thoracic vertebrae through a spinal branch that enters through the intervertebral foramen.

The spinal cord and its coverings (meninges) are located in the vertebral canal of the thoracic spine. The thoracic spine contains the thoracic and upper lumbar spinal cord segments along with their anterior and posterior nerve roots. Thoracic spinal nerves (12 pairs) are formed just outside the intervertebral foramen by the union of the anterior and posterior roots. In the thoracic spine, the spinal nerves are formed below the vertebra they correspond to in number. Thus, the T1 spinal nerve is formed just outside the intervertebral foramen between the T1 and T2 vertebrae. After the spinal nerve is formed, it divides almost immediately into anterior and posterior primary rami. The posterior primary rami innervate segmentally skin and muscles of the back as well as the zygapophyseal joints of the thoracic spine. The anterior primary rami enter the intercostal spaces and become the intercostal nerves innervating segmentally skin and muscles of the anterolateral thoracic and abdominal walls. Situated on the anterior aspect of the necks of the ribs, on each side of the thoracic spine, are the thoracic sympathetic trunks consisting of 11 to12 ganglia linked together. Each ganglion is connected to an intercostal nerve by two branches. The last ganglion may be connected to both the eleventh and twelfth intercostal nerves. Arising from the ganglia of the thoracic sympathetic trunks are three splanchnic nerves (greater, lesser, and least), which descend toward the diaphragm on the anterior aspects of the thoracic vertebral bodies.

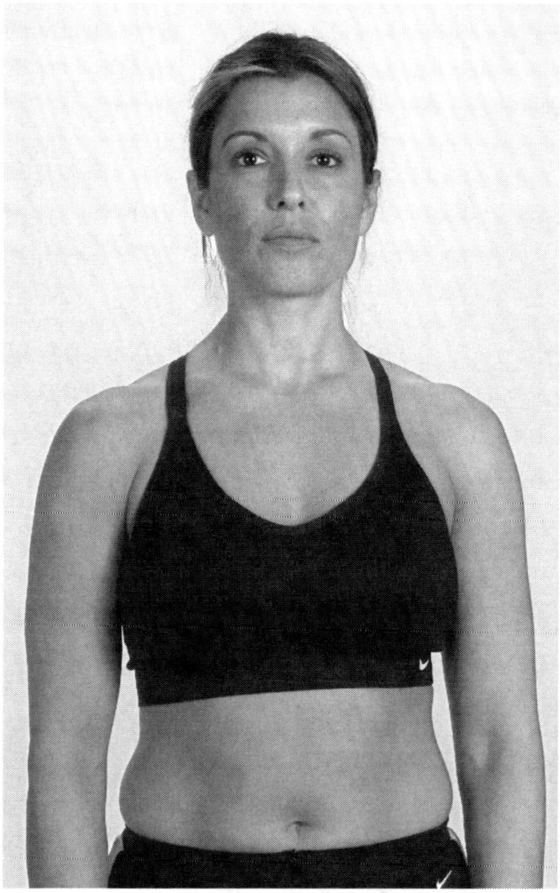

Figure 5.1. Observe the patient's posture from the front.

PHYSICAL EXAMINATION

Observation

The examiner should be situated directly in front of the patient, standing far enough away to view the entire body so that posture can be assessed (Figure 5.1). Assessment begins by noting the appearance of the spine and related structures.

Observe the patient's posture, both in a seated and standing position. Note any obvious deformities, such as asymmetry on either side of the spine (Figure 5.2) or in an anterior-posterior view (Figure 5.3), keeping in mind the relationship the thorax has with the truck and axial skeleton.

The areas of the thoracic spine generate power for the lower extremities and stability for the upper extremities. These principles of observation are key for patients who develop instability patterns, for the dysfunction and its cause may not always be in the same place.

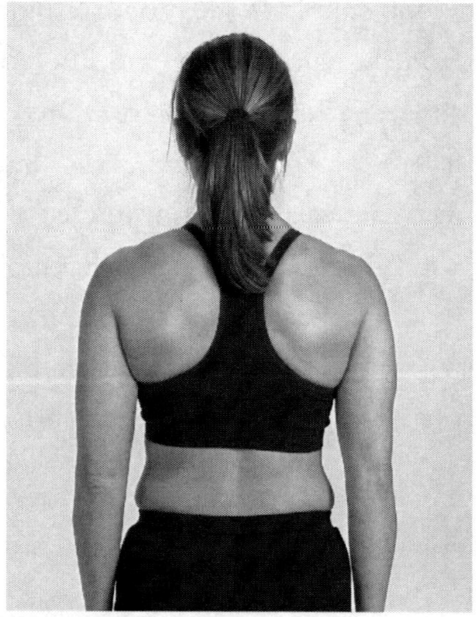

Figure 5.2. Observe spine posteriorly.

Look at the chest wall and determine if there is right-to-left symmetry. Note any abnormalities such as pectus excavatum (funnel chest), pecutus carinatum (pigeon chest), or barrel chest, which may be related to an underlying medical problem. From the side, observe the anterior-posterior diameter for an increased or decrease, and note the right versus the left. From the posterior aspect, note the symmetry from one side of the spine to the other, any curvatures to the spine, any "fullness" of the musculature, or any skin problems, such as rashes or moles. The patient should first be examined in a standing position, to assess normal posture, then in the seated position, to note any "slumping" or bending of the torso, indicating either poor posture or abnormalities of the musculature or spine itself. Correlate any finding with the rest of the evaluation in determining the correct diagnosis and associated treatment.

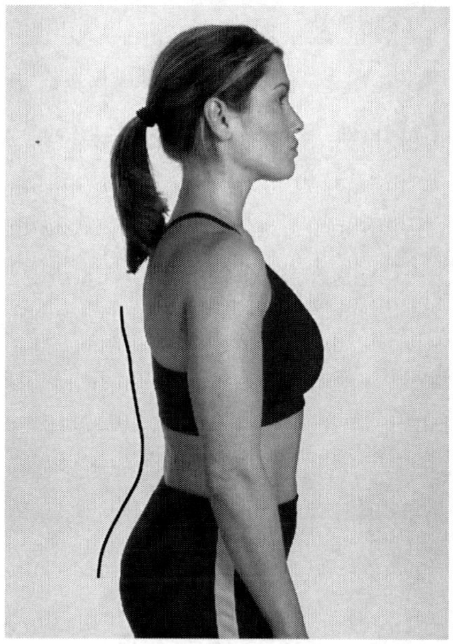

Figure 5.3. Lateral view of the spine.

Palpation

Begin with the patient standing. Place the finger pads along the spine, first over the spinous processes, then the transverse processes, and finally over the paraspinal muscles. Feel for tissue texture changes, asymmetry of landmarks, restriction of motion, and tenderness to palpation.

When evaluating the patient, it is possible to find areas of tenderness while palpating along the spine, which are related

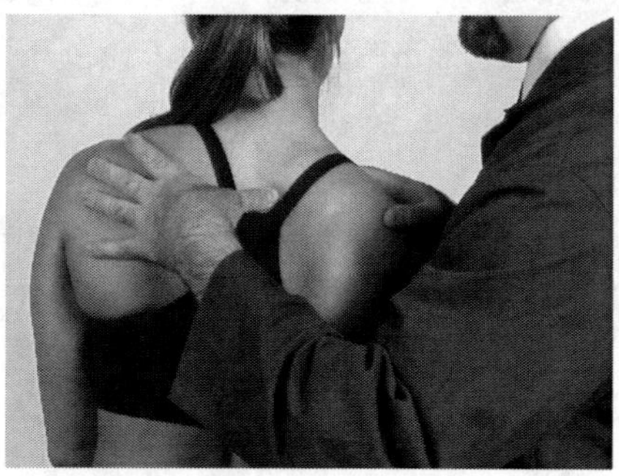

Figure 5.4. Passive motion testing of the thoracic spine.

to muscles that are in spasm. In considering the diagnosis of a tender point, it is helpful to know where tender points are most common. They may be located posteriorly or anteriorly. Posterior points are found while examining the patient's back, and may be located either on the tip of the lateral surface of the spinous process, or at the tip of the transverse process. Anterior points are found when examining the patient's front, while assessing the rib cage and other pertinent areas related to the thoracic spine.

Often, a tender point along the costovertebral junction in the thoracic spine will lead to a tender point on the corresponding anterior sternochondral junction. For instance, a patient with a tender left T5 dysfunction will likely have a tender point at the left fifth sternochondral junction anteriorly; i.e., a dysfunction at one end of the rib attachment leads to dysfunction at the other end.

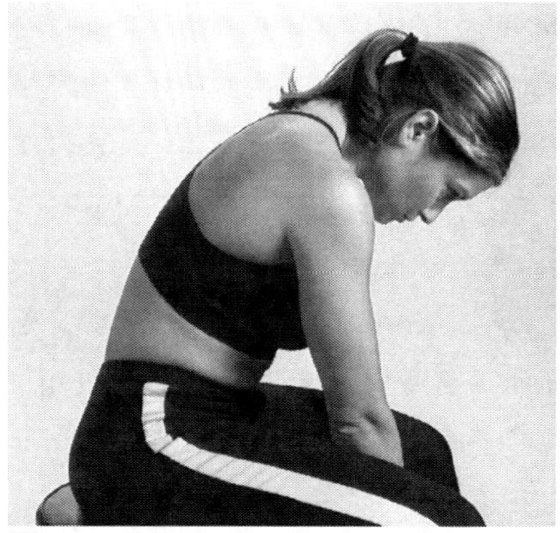

Figure 5.5. Active flexion of the thoracic spine.

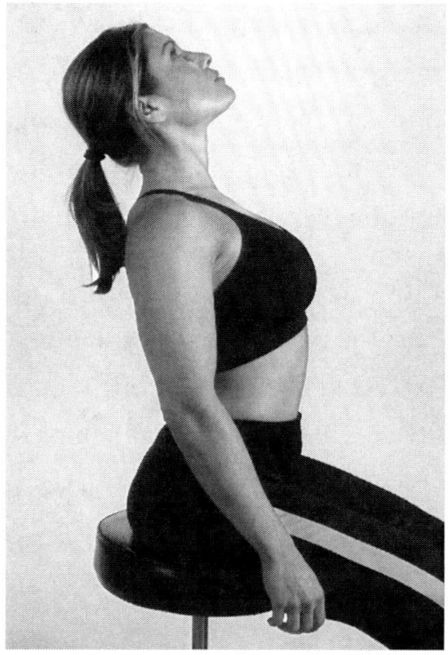

Figure 5.6. Active extension of the thoracic spine.

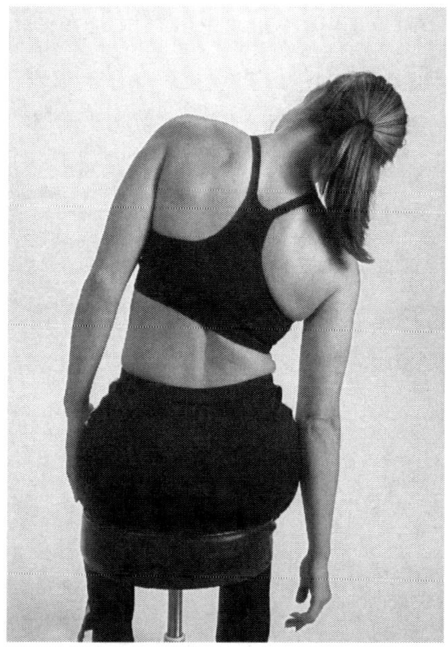

Figure 5.7. Active side-bending of the thoracic spine.

Motion Testing

Gross Active and Passive Range of Motion

To test passive motion, the patient sits in a "natural" seated posture. The examiner places one thumb on the patient's uppermost thoracic transverse process on the side being evaluated and the other hand over the acromion, cupping the shoulder with the web of his or her hand, and inducing the appropriate motion (Figure 5.4). The examiner's body can be placed against the patient's back to isolate the thoracic spine and block out accessory movement created by the lumber spine, cervical spine, or extremities.

Active range of motion can be assessed by asking the patient to slump over (flexion) (Figure 5.5), arch the back as far as the patient can (extension) (Figure 5.6), and side-bend with the arms to the side (Figure 5.7), either sitting or standing. Rotating the upper torso would be enough to judge thoracic rotation (Figure 5.8).

Segmental Motion Testing

While the patient is seated, the examiner tests the spine for TART findings, as done for palpation. Next, examine flexion and extension. Place the finders in the interspinal spaces and feel for changes, or gaps, as you flex or extend at that segment. Gaps widen in flexion and narrow in extension. Note any asymmetry among levels. For side bending and rotation motion, place the pads of your second and third fingers on either side of the specific spinous process, and note changes or gaps as motion is induced.

To examine the upper spine (T1-T6) move the patient's head in the direction you want the spine to move (Figure 5.9). To examine the lower spine, grasp the patient's shoulder opposite the segment you are palpating and move the patient's body appropriately for each motion test (Figure 5.10).

Move the patient to the prone position, which puts the thoracic spine in neutral position. To test in flexion, the patient curls up into a "catlike" position, with the hips raised in the air (Figure 5.11). For extension, the patient arches his or her back while leaning on the elbows (this is sometimes referred to as the "sphinx" position) (Figure 5.12).

In each of the above positions, side bending and rotation are monitored by palpating the intersegmental spaces as mentioned previously, and by pressing on the transverse processes, posteriorly to anteriorly. If there is resistance, tenderness to palpation, or pain at the site, then there is a dysfunction at the segment. For example, if a patient is in the sphinx position (extension) and the transverse process of T8 on the left is tender and difficult to push toward the right, it is diagnosed as T8 extension, rotated left, side-bent left, per Fryette's second principle.

Scoliosis

Scoliosis is an abnormal lateral curvature to the spine, but it can also extend to the cervical and

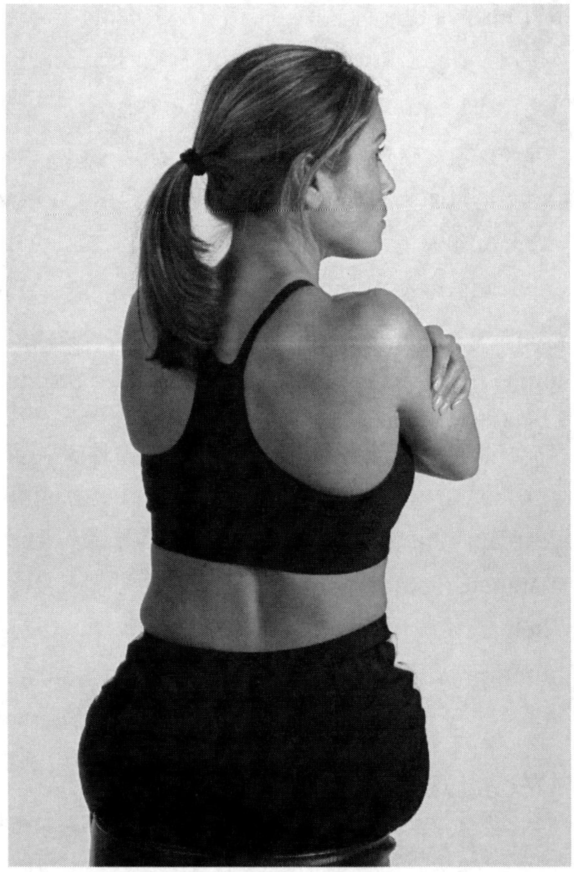

Figure 5.8. Active rotation of the thoracic spine (patient should be seated).

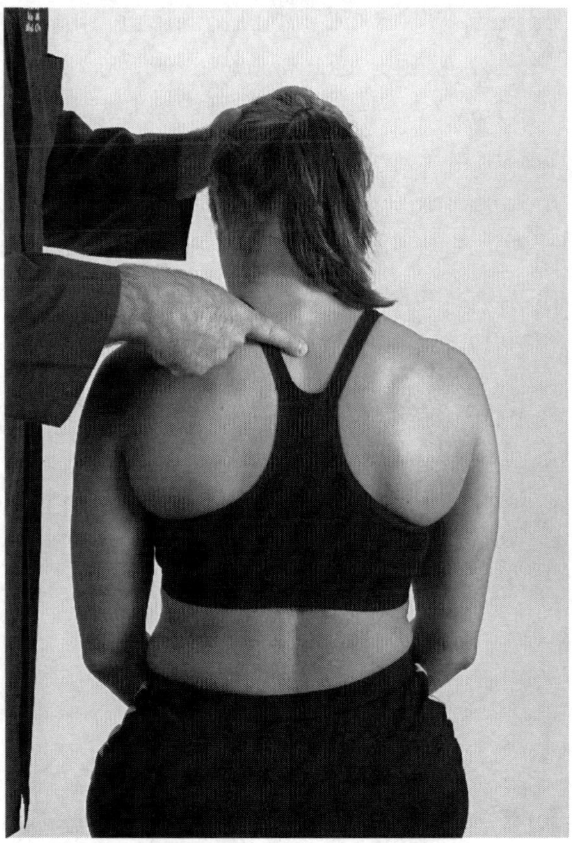

Figure 5.9. Exam of upper thoracic spine.

lumbar areas in varying degrees. Scoliosis is diagnosed most often in adolescence due to the rapid growth spurt, which makes this condition more noticeable. The causes may be structural or nonstructural. Structural changes can involve genetic, idiopathic, or congenital problems of vertebral formation, or loss of flexibility. Nonstructural changes can involve poor posture, inflammation, nerve root irritation, leg-length discrepancy, or hip contracture. Scoliosis is classified by the curve pattern found, which is designated according to the level of the apex of the curve. For example, a left thoracic curve would have a convexity toward the left, where the apex sits.

When palpating the spine, note any muscle spasms and changes in the bony and soft tissue contours on either side, as well as any abnormalities of the ribs, either in position or during motion. The patient should be examined in standing and seated positions, noting any postural deficiencies, such as slouching in the chair or not standing straight. Look at the posterior spine as the patient bends forward to touch his or her toes (Figure 5.13). Also note changes from left to right, and superior to inferior, as you view the entire body, especially the tips of the ears, shoulders (specifically the tip of the acromion process), scapulae, and hips (iliac crest).

The pathologic process that occurs with scoliosis may have long-lasting clinical impact on the patient, so prompt recognition and treatment are important. Primary thoracic scoliosis carries the worst prognosis of any type because of its rapid progression and the severity of associated clinical deformities. When there is evidence of a structural scoliosis, the spine appears distorted from the vertebral bodies

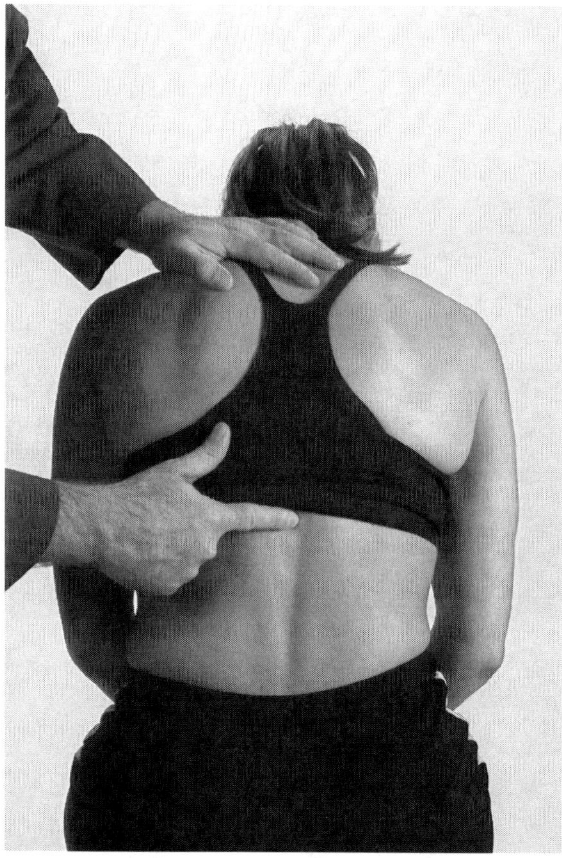

Figure 5.10. Exam of lower thoracic spine.

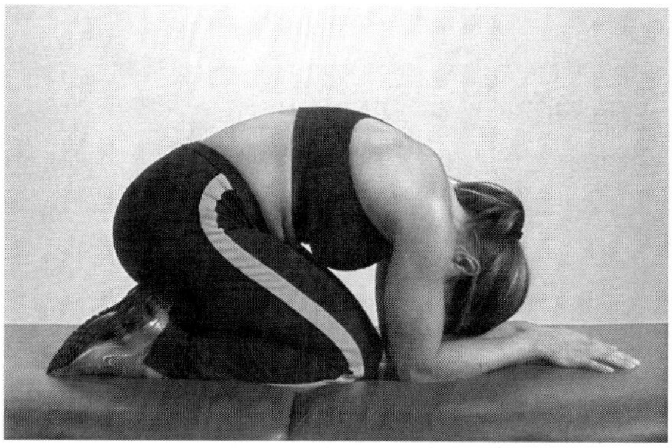

Figure 5.11. Testing segmental motion in flexion.

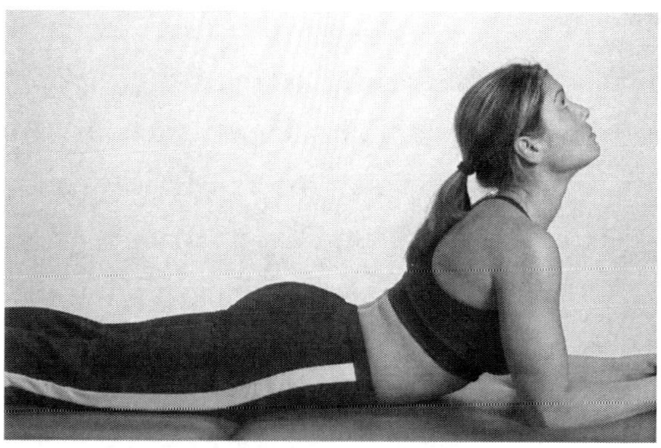

Figure 5.12. Testing segmental motionin extension.

rotation to the convex side, and this pushes the ipsilateral ribs posteriorly—causing a "hump"—while narrowing the thoracic cage on the ipsilateral side. The spinous processes deviate toward the concave side, shifting the ipsilateral ribs anteriorly—causing a "hollow"—while widening the thoracic cage on the contralateral side. These changes can decrease the surface area under the thoracic cage. This can result in respiratory and cardiac problems, such as increased intrathoracic pressure and decreased compliance of the lungs. Severe cases can even cause compression of the vascular structures. The body always tries to compensate for the scoliosis in order to deep the eyes balanced and level with the horizon. This results in changes to the spine, hips, and legs, which may exacerbate pain and other medical conditions.

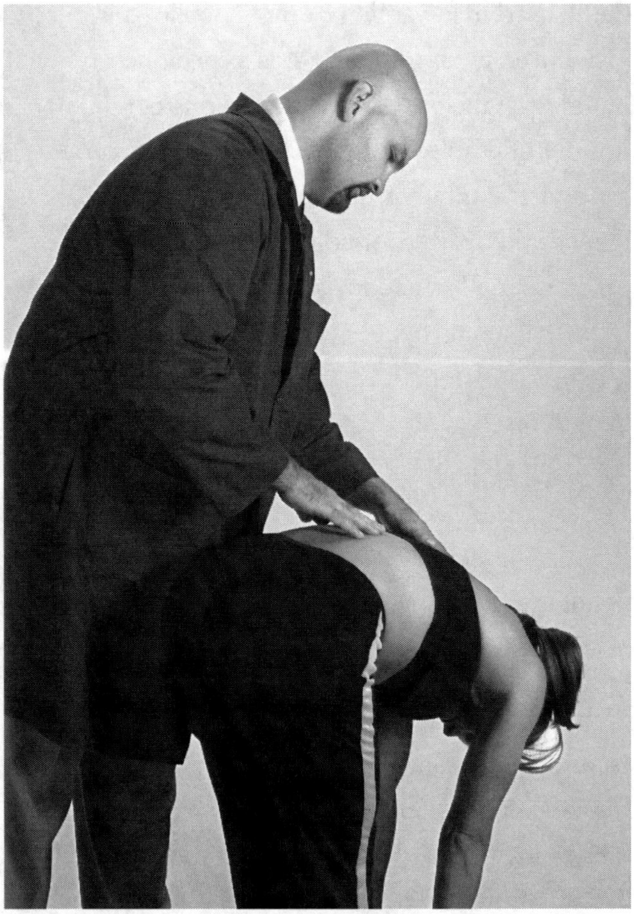

Figure 5.13. Observe thoracic spine from behind with patient moving from upright to fully flexed forward.

Scapular Dysfunction

The scapula is an important structure because of its relationship to the thoracic spine. With its muscular attachments to the spine and the rib cage, motion about the spine can be inhibited by dysfunction of either scapula. On appearance, both scapulae should be equidistant from the spine and at equal height, without deviation, including any abduction or adduction. Also, note if one side appears "winged," which would look like a bird with an injured wing that hangs to the side. This condition may be due to long thoracic nerve palsy or weakness of the serratus anterior muscle. Sprengel's deformity occurs when one scapula is congenitally elevated and possibly atrophied, or smaller than the other.

When physically examining the scapula, palpate along the superior, medial, and lateral borders of the bone. The scapular spine is felt just beneath the acromion, and sits at the level of the third thoracic spinous process. Medially and superiorly, moving downward along the edge of the scapula, feel for any muscle changes (this is the levator scapulae area), such as tender points or tissue texture changes. The medial border should be parallel to the spine and sit about 5 cm lateral to the vertebrae. The inferior angle of the medial border sits at the level of the seventh thoracic spinous process (Figure 5.14).

If the scapula is winged, you may appreciate the medial border coming off the rib cage instead of sitting flat against it, as expected in a normal scapula. The lateral border, which is harder to palpate than the medial due to multiple muscle attachments, should be palpated moving from the inferomedial to the superolateral edge.

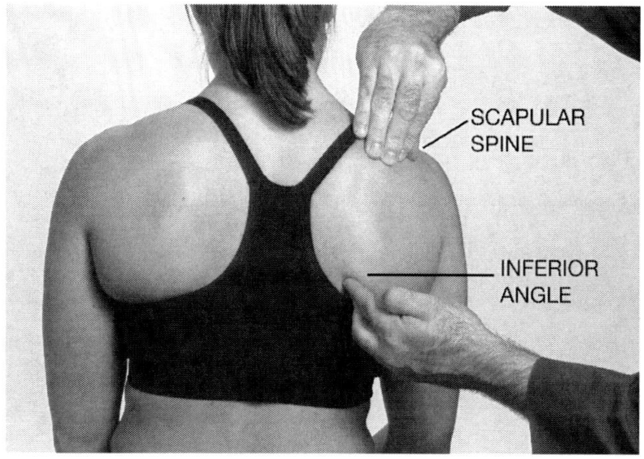

Figure 5.14. Scapular landmarks.

Rib Cage

The thoracic spine has articulation with the rib cage posteriorly, and any dysfunction of the ribs can affect the spine to various degrees. Often a rib dysfunction will cause or correspond with a thoracic dysfunction at the same level. Conditions such as scoliosis affect the ribs in terms of position and motion. Because of the ribs' association with the lungs, rib abnormalities can result in altered respiratory mechanics.

The ribs should be palpated individually and as a group, noting asymmetry, difference in space between the ribs on one side compared with the other, and tissue texture changes. Having the patient inhale and exhale allows the examiner to assess the motion of the ribs. Keep in mind the rules of rib motion: ribs 1 to 5 exhibit primarily "pump-handle" motion, whereas ribs 6 to 10 exhibit primarily "bucket-handle" motion. Ribs 11 and 12, which do not articulate with the thoracic cage, undergo caliper motion. Pump-handle rib motion is best palpated by placing the ulnar side of your hand on the patient's rib cage anterorly and laterally to the sternum. Bucket-handle motion is best palpated by placing your hands, with fingers pointed laterally, on the anterior rib cage, just below the level of the sternum. Caliper motion is appreciated by putting your hands on the anterior-inferiormost portion of the rib cage, again with fingers pointing outward, and monitoring the ribs as the patient inhales and exhales.

The first and second ribs are best monitored with finger pads in the first intercostal space. First rib pump-handle contacts are against the inferior rib margin on either side of the manubrium, while the bucket-handle contact is lateral at a point where the rib passes under the clavicle. The other ribs have pump-handle contacts at the costochondral margins. The other bucket-handle contact points are along the rib shafts in the midaxillary line.

Rib Motion Testing

The patient can be supine or sitting, although a sitting patient allows the examiner to flex and extend the spine. The examiner places both hands on the chest wall, checking three areas:

1. Anterior upper bucket-handle motion (Figure 5.15).
2. Anterior middle pump-handle motion (Figure 5.16).
3. Posterior rib angles (Figure 5.17).

In each case, the fingers lightly touch the ribs and follow their motion through inspiration and expiration and compare for asymmetry.

Floating Ribs

The patient is best examined prone, as the examiner places his or her hands on the lumbar paravertebral and flank region. Sliding the skin up, down, and in circles will unveil the twelfth rib shafts. Allow the ribs to move your hands and follow the hand movement; there is no need for the hands to change positions. Check for symmetry.

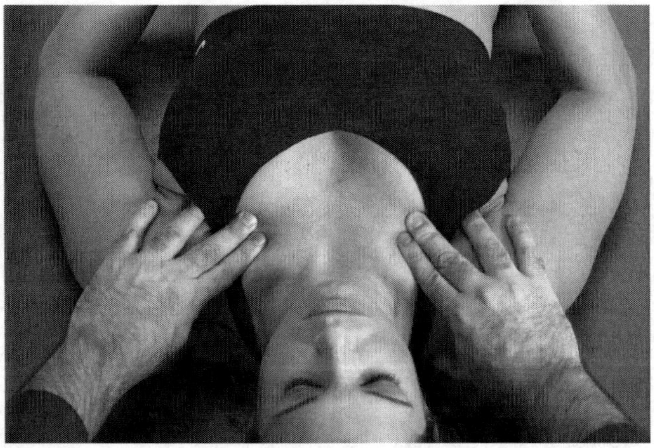

Figure 5.15. Anterior upper bucket-handle type motion.

Neurovascular Examination

In the thoracic spine, there are no specific superficial or deep tendon reflexes to indicate nerve root problems. However, there is a great deal of association between sympathetic reflexes and dermatomes (or cutaneous reflexes) and thoracic spine dysfunction.

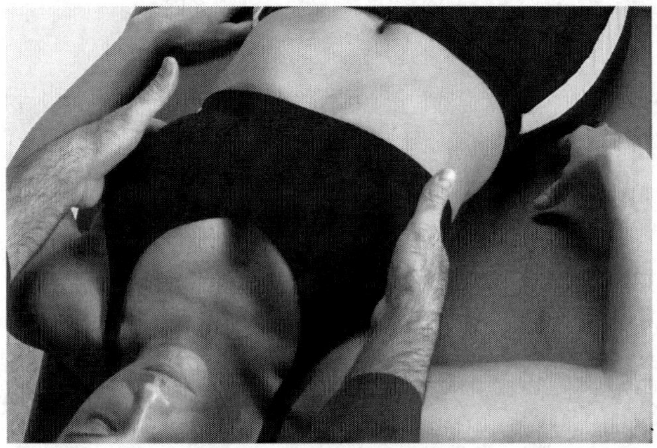

Figure 5.16. Anterior middle ribs pump-handle type motion.

Dermatomes

The dermatomes that are supplied by the thoracic nerve roots follow the pattern of the ribs. The anatomic arrangement of the neurovascular bundle is known by the acronym VAN (Vein Artery Nerve), and it runs along the inferior edge of the rib body. Dermatomes represent cutaneous branches of the dorsal and ventral rami, and each spinal nerve innervates a continuous strip of skin that extends from the posterior midline to the anterior midline. There is much overlapping of segments in the thoracic region, where one dermatome may be in the same area as the next.

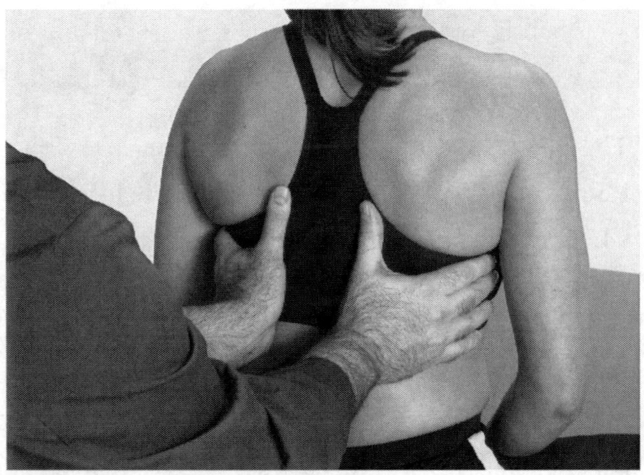

Figure 5.17. Posterior rib angles.

Note any lesion or pathology that follows a dermatomal pattern. One such disorder of clinical significance is Herpes zoster (shingles), which is a viral infection that is embedded in the spinal nerve ganglia. Herpes zoster causes sharp, burning pain in a dermatomal distribution of the nerve it infects, followed shortly after by an erythematous (red) vesicular rash. It usually sits in only one dermatome unilaterally without crossing over the midline.

Sympathetic Reflexes

A somatic dysfunction in the thoracic spine may sometimes correlate with a clinical finding or pathology from a visceral structure. Sympathethic innervations that arise from the thoracic rami supply various organs in the body, and when there is a problem with one of these organs, a viscerosomatic reflex may occur between an organ and the spine (via the nerve pathway).

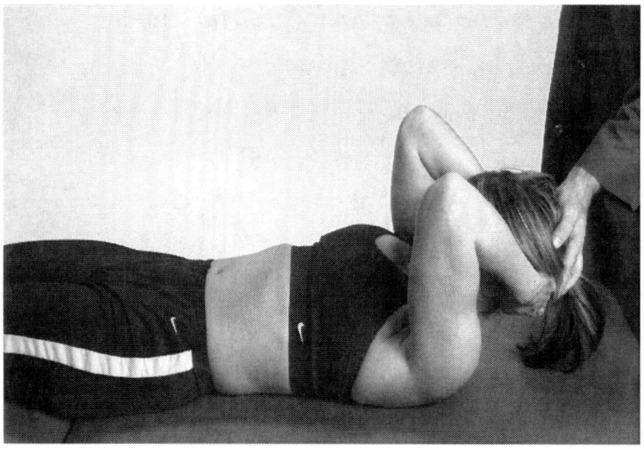

Figure 5.18. Brudzinski's Test.

PROVOCATIVE TEST AND MANEUVERS

Brudzinski's/Kernig's Test - BASIC EXAM. With the patient supine and the hands behind the head, he or she flexes the head onto the chest ***(Brudzinski's Test)*** (Figure 5.18) and/or flexes the hip with an extended knee ***(Kernig's Test)*** (Figure 5.19).

> *Positive Test*: Pain or stiffness of the head, neck, or low back.
>
> *Indicates*: Meningeal irritation, nerve root problems, or dural irritation.

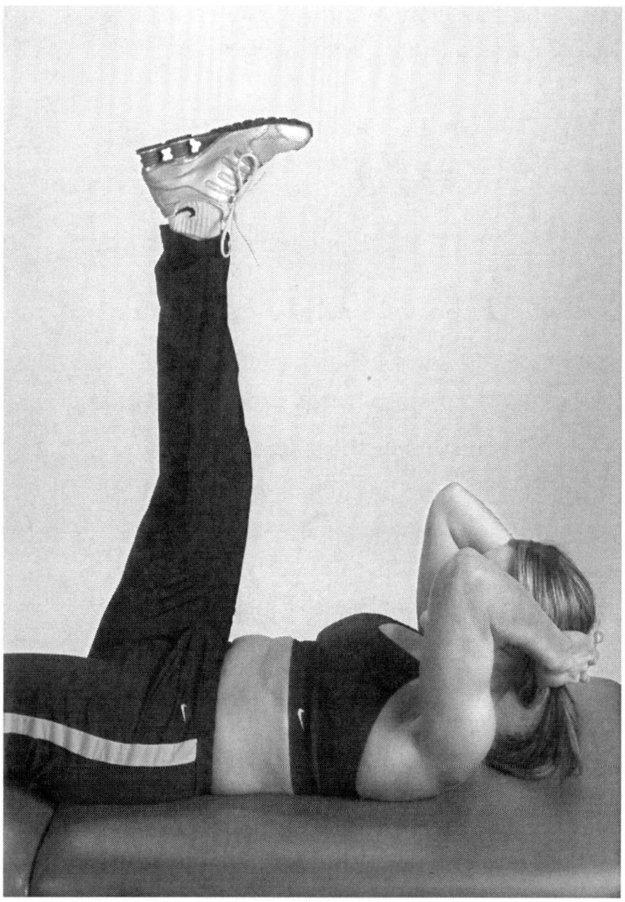

Figure 5.19. Kernig's Test.

Sitting Dural Stretch Test (Slump Test). The seated patient "slumps" forward with the shoulders sagging and the spine flexed. The examiner flexes the neck of the patient, then passively extends one knee to 0 degrees (Figure 5.20).

> *Positive Test*: Pain on the ipsilateral side at the site of the dysfunction.
>
> *Indicates*: Impingement of the dura and spinal cord or nerve root.

First Thoracic Nerve Root Stretch. The seated patient abducts the arm 90 degrees and flexes the pronated forearm 90 degrees. The examiner puts the patient's hand behind the neck (Figure 5.21).

Positive Test: Pain in the scapular area or the arm.

Indicates: First thoracic nerve injury, ulnar nerve injury.

Passive Scapular Approximation. The examiner has the patient lying prone on the table and passively lifts the patient's shoulder (scapula) up and back (Figure 5.22).

Positive Test: Pain in the ipsilateral scapular area.

Indicates: T1 and T2 neural impingement.

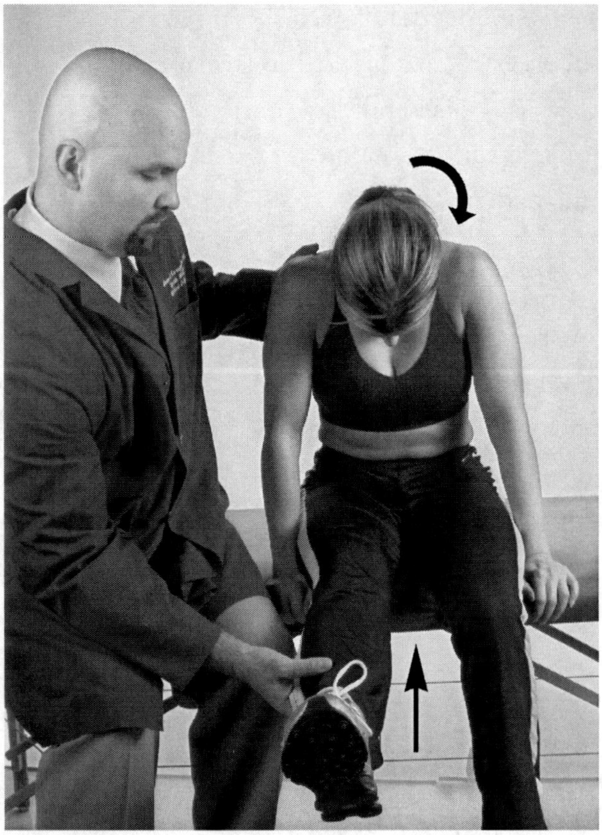

Figure 5.20. The Slump Test.

Scapular Elevation - BASIC EXAM. The examiner stands behind the standing patient and places his or her hands on each acromion. With arms resting at the side, the patient shrugs his or her shoulders against examiner resistance (Figure 5.23).

Positive Test: Weakness or pain against resistance.

Indicates: Tendonitis (of trapezius and/or levator scapulae muscles), cervical injury, or cranial nerve damage (spinal accessory nerve, CN XI).

Scapular Retraction. The patient stands with his or her arm adducted and the elbow slightly bent. The examiner stands behind the patient, cupping his or her hand on the ipsilateral elbow, and has the patient resist as the examiner abducts the scapula (Figure 5.24).

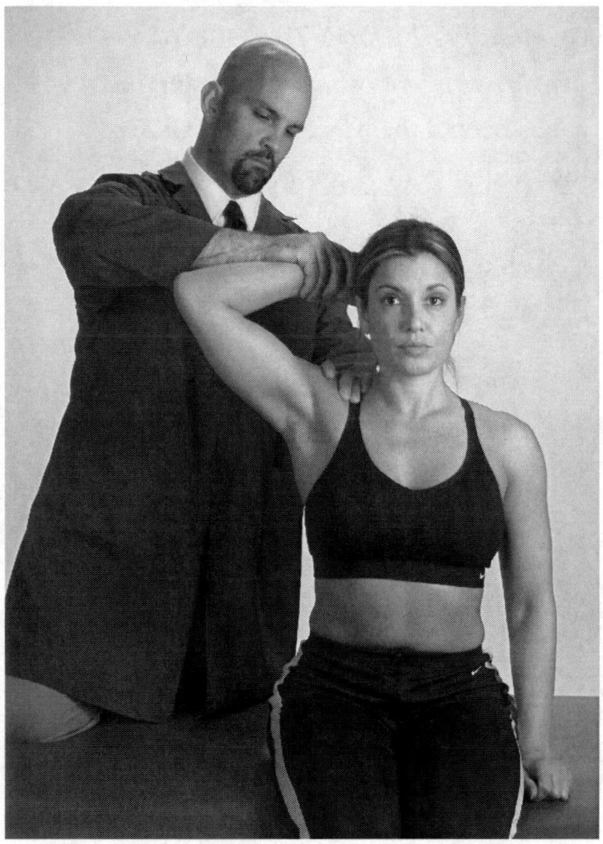

Figure 5.21. First thoracic nerve root stretch.

Positive Test: Painful or weak response during resistance.

Indicates: Rhomboids and/or trapezius dysfunction, thoracic spinal dysfunction.

Scapular Protraction (Winging) - BASIC EXAM. The examiner stands behind the upright patient, whose arm is flexed forward with elbow bent, both at 90 degrees, and places one hand over the thoracic spine for stabilization. The other hand grasps the proximal aspect of the patient's forearm and attempts to pull the arm backward, while the patient resists by moving the arm forward (Figure 5.25).

Alternate maneuver: The patient pushes against a wall with both hands with the feet farther away from the wall than the shoulder.

Positive Test: Scapular winging, pain, and/or weakness during maneuvers.

Indicates: Serratus anterior muscle weakness. Lower trapezius dysfunction may result in the medial winging of the scapula, partly because the trapezius muscle maintains the medial scapular border close to the vertebral column.

THORACIC OUTLET SYNDROME PROVOCATIVE TESTS

Elevated Arm Stress Test (EAST) or "Hands-up" Test. The patient externally rotates the shoulders with the elbows slightly behind the head. The patient then opens and closes his or her hands slowly for 3 minutes (Figure 5.26).

Positive Test: Pain, heaviness, or profound arm weakness or numbness and tingling of the hand.

Indicates: Thoracic outlet syndrome.

Costoclavicular Test. The examiner monitors the

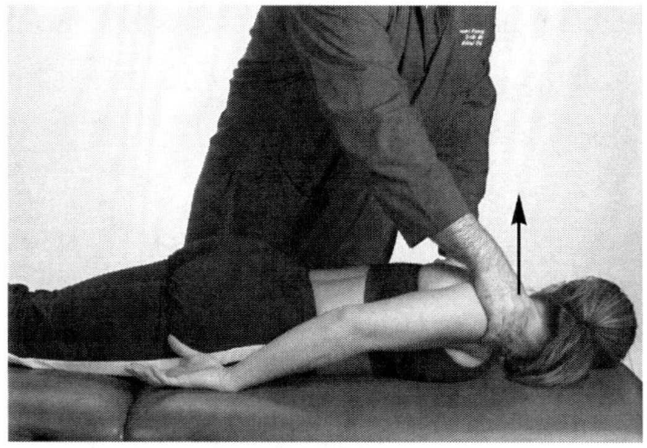

Figure 5.22. Passive scapular approximation.

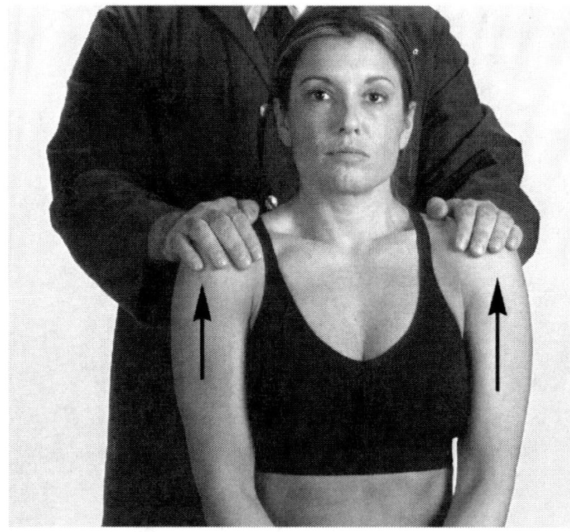

Figure 5.23. Active scapular elevation.

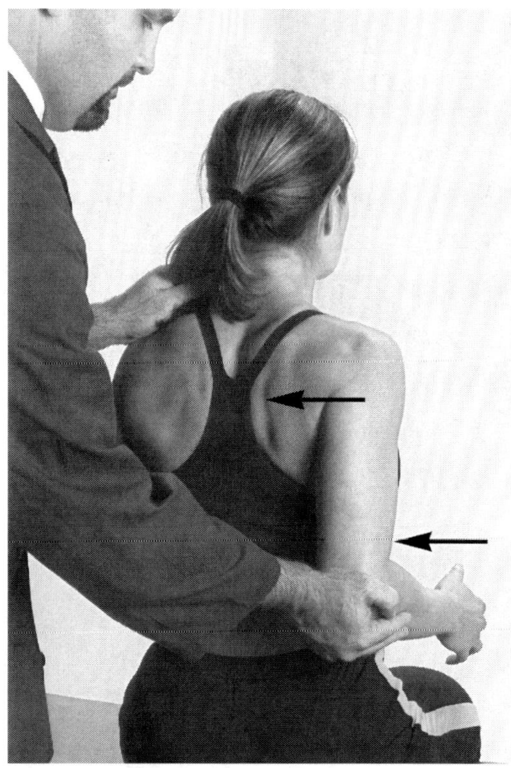

Figure 5.24. Scapular retraction.

radial pulse. The examiner draws the shoulder down and back as the patient assumes a "military" posture (chest out) (Figure 5.27).

Positive Test: Disappearance or diminution of the pulse, or if the symptoms are elicited.

Indicates: Thoracic outlet syndrome, usually due to compression of the subclavian neurovascular bundle by the clavicle.

Adson's Test - BASIC EXAM. The examiner abducts the patient's affected arm to 90 degrees and palpates the radial pulse. The patient is instructed to turn his or her head toward the affected side and take a deep inhalation (Figure 5.28).

Positive Test: The disappearance or diminution of the pulse or provocation of symptoms.

Indicates: Thoracic outlet syndrome, usually related to the scalene musculature.

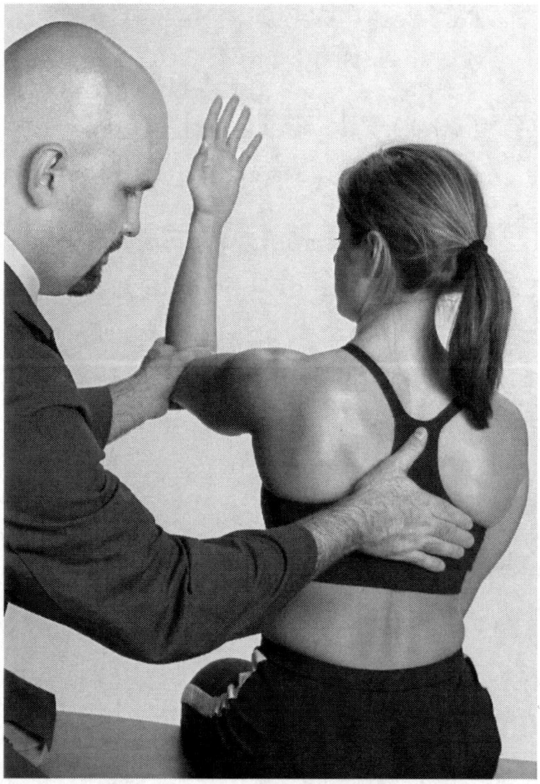

Figure 5.25. Scapular protraction.

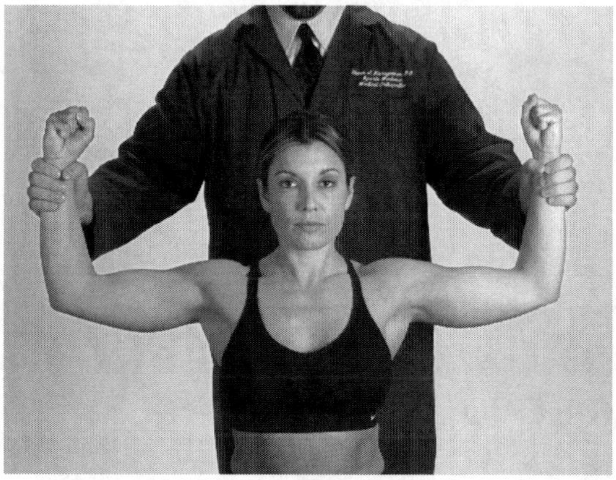

Figure 5.26. Elevated Arm Stress Test.

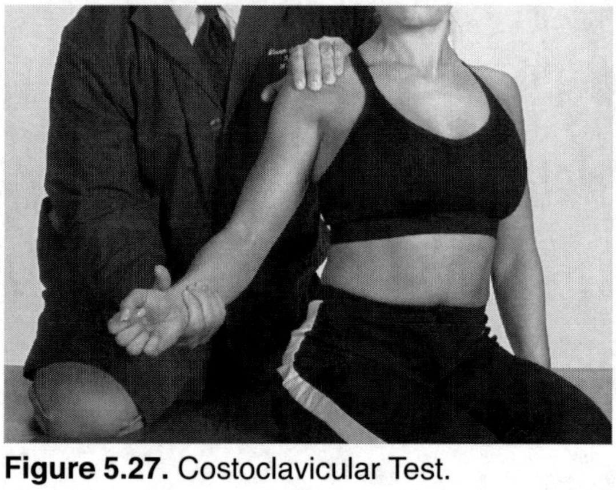

Figure 5.27. Costoclavicular Test.

COMMON CONDITIONS

- Thoracic outlet syndrome
- Thoracic somatic dysfunction
- First rib somatic dysfunction
- Rib somatic dysfunction
- Scapular elevation/protraction/retraction
- Thoracic spine compression fractures
- Scoliosis
- Facet hypertrophy/arthropathy

CONDITIONS THAT SHOULD NOT BE MISSED DUE TO MORBIDITY AND/ OR MORTALITY

- Nuchal rigidity (meningitis)
- Displaced/dislocated thoracic spine fractures
- Tumors

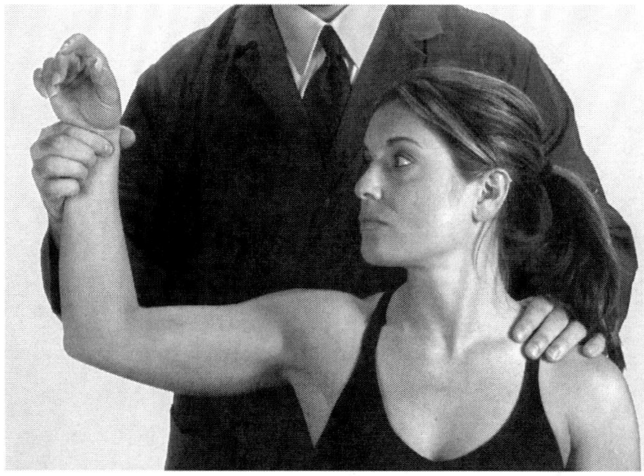

Figure 5.28. Adson's Test.

REFERENCES

1. Karageanes SJ. *Principles of Manual Sports Medicine.* Philadelphia, PA: Lippincott Williams & Wilkins; 2005; p. 263-282.

6 The Lumbar Spine Exam

Charles W. Webb, D.O.

Shawn Kerger, D.O.

Of the entire human body, the physical examination of the lumbar spine could be the most important examination to know and fully understand. Nearly two thirds of adults will experience low back pain in their lifetime.[1] It is so common that only symptoms of an upper respiratory infection present to primary care physicians more than low back pain.[2] Of all the physician visits a year, it is the fifth most common reason.[2] With this extraordinary data, one can easily understand the magnitude of this problem on society in terms of pain and the financial burden. In fact, the direct costs in diagnosing and treatment of low back pain were estimated to be $25 billion annually in the United States.[3]

Like the entire body, the lower back has multiple anatomical structures that are intricately connected in a fascinating way to allow us to lift objects twice our weight, hit a baseball or simply bend over to tie your shoes. One must make continuous effort to remember this in examination of the lumbar spine. One can easily envision how dysfunctions of the quadratus lumborum, facet joints and lumbar vertebrae can cause dysfunction in this region. But, it's the connections through fascia and ligaments that also allow for dysfunctions of the shoulder, pelvis and legs to indirectly lead to somatic complaints of the lumbosacral spine. During the examination, you will be using information from your history to make your diagnosis.

Knowing that the vast majority of somatic complaints are musculoskeletal in origin is crucial. However, a physician must not become nearsighted and forget other sources of lumbosacral complaints. The history should always precede the examination and this allows the elimination of serious pathology included in the differential of low back pain. Excluding "red flags" such as fevers, incontinence, night pain, weight loss, steroid use, parenteral drug abuse, migrating cramping pain or a history of cancer will aid in the exclusion of infection, cauda equina syndrome (CES), fracture, nephrolithiasis and malignancy.

APPLIED ANATOMY AND BIOMECHANICS

The motion segment of the lumbar spine consists of an intervertebral disc located between adjacent vetebral bodies and 2 zygapophyseal (facet) joints. The intervertebral disc is composed of the nucleus pulposus and the annulus fibrosis. The nucleus pulposus is made up of fibrocartilage, whose water binding capacity decreases with age, causing degenerative changes (spondylosis) to start after the second decade of life. Initially the disc is 85-90% water, but will decrease to approximately 65% with age.

The annulus fibrosis is a fibro cartilage that is composed of 20 concentric rings of collagenous fibers that crisscross each other to accommodate torsional movements. The facet joints are non-weight-bearing joints, located on the vertebral arches with the superior facets facing posteromedial and the inferior facets facing anterolateral. Disc degeneration (spondylosis) transfers the weight bearing to the facet joints and may produce inflammation, arthropathy, and increased force upon the disc leading to herniation.[4]

The discs are avascular with only the periphery receiving a blood supply. The disc does not have a nerve supply. The pain sensitive structures around the disc are the anterior longitudinal ligament, posterior longitudinal ligament, vertebral body, nerve root, and the cartilage of the facet joint. Nerve roots exit through relatively large intervertebral foramina and each one is named for the vertebra above it. (Example, L4 nerve root exits between the L4 and the L5 vertebrae.) The L4 disc is between the L4 and the L5 vertebrae (Figure 6.1). Because of this arrangement and the course of the nerve root, the L4 disc only rarely compresses the L4 nerve root; it is more likely to compress the L5 nerve root. The L5 and S1 segment is the most common site of problems in the vertebral column because this level bears more weight than any other level.

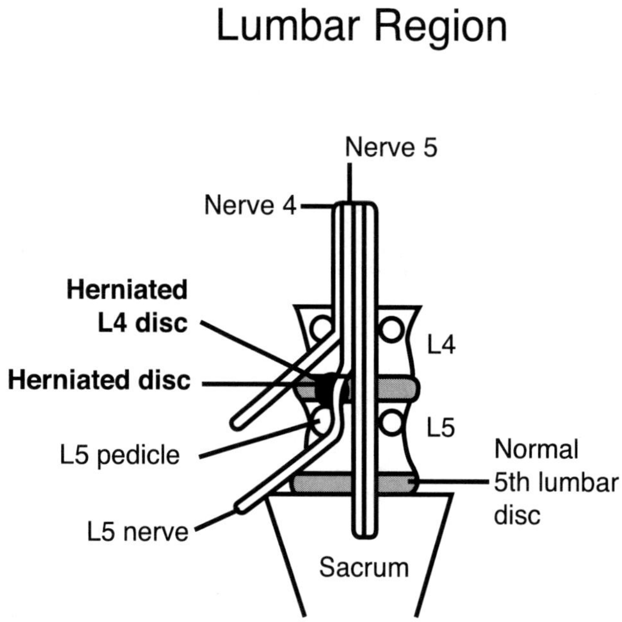

Figure 6.1. Relationship of discs and exiting nerve roots in the lumbar spine.

There are two muscular support groups of the lumbar spine. The Psoas and the abdominal muscles comprise the anterior group, and the posterior group is made up of the superficial, middle, and deep layers of the paraspinal muscles. The superficial layer is made up of the erector spinea (iliocostalis, longissimus, and spinalis). These function as the chief extensors of the vertebral column. The middle layer is the multifidi muscles and the deep layer consists of small inter-segmental muscles.[4]

The major motion planes of the lumbar spine are flexion (forward bending), extension (backward bending), side bending, and rotation. Flexion and extension occur mainly at the lower two segments whereas rotation at each lumbar segment is limited to only a few degrees secondary to the position of the facet joints. Movements that combine flexion and rotation have the highest injury potential.[4]

PHYSICAL EXAMINATION

History

All patients, with acute LBP should be risk stratified with an initial assessment attempting to identify "red flag" (Table 6.1) responses or findings in the history and physical examination that indicate a potentially serious underlying condition, such as a fracture, tumor, infection, abdominal aneurysm, or CES, that can lead to considerable patient morbidity and/or mortality. These clinical clues (red flags) include a history of major trauma, minor trauma in patients older than 50 years of age, persistent fever, history of cancer, metabolic disorder, major muscle weakness, bladder or bowel dysfunction, saddle anesthesia, decreased sphincter tone, and unrelenting night pain. Red flags stratify the patient to an increased risk and should prompt an earlier clinical action, such as imaging or laboratory work up.

Table 6.1. Red Flags and Appropriate Actions

Condition	Red Flag	Action
Cancer	*History of Cancer *Unexplained weight loss *Age ≥ 50 *Failure to improve with therapy *Pain ≥ 4-6 weeks *Night/rest pain	If malignant disease of the spine is suspected, imaging is indicated and CBC, ESR, should be considered. Identification of possible primary malignancy should be investigated, e.g., PSA, mammogram, UPEP/SPEP/IPEP
Infection	*Fever *History of intravenous drug use *Recent bacterial infection: UTI, skin, pneumonia *Immunocompromised states (steroid, organ transplants, diabetes, HIV) *Rest pain	If infection in the spine is suspected, MRI, CBC, ESR and/or UA are indicated
Cauda Equina Syndrome	*Urinary retention or incontinence *Saddle anesthesia *Anal sphincter tone decrease/ fecal incontinence *Bilateral lower extremity weakness/ numbness or progressive neurological deficit	Request immediate surgical consultation
Fracture	*Use of corticosteroids *Age ≥ 70 or history of osteoporosis *Recent significant trauma	Appropriate imaging and surgical consultation
Acute Abdominal Aneurysm	*Abdominal pulsating mass *Other atherosclerotic vascular disease *Rest/night pain *Age ≥ 60	Appropriate imaging (ultrasound) and surgical consultation
Significant Herniated Nucleus Pulposus (HNP)	Major muscle weakness	Appropriate imaging and surgical consultation

Psychosocial factors also significantly affect pain and function in LBP patients. These psychosocial factors are known as "yellow flags" (Table 6.2) and are better predictors of treatment outcomes than physical factors in some patients.

Observation

The examination of the lumbar spine begins with a visual inspection. Ideally the patient will be wearing clothing that allows for full examination, such as shorts and a sports bra. First look for any specific posturing: patients holding themselves in an antalgic way will lend support to

Table 6.2. Yellow Flags in Low Back Pain

Belief Systems	Co-morbid Conditions
-Fear Avoidance -Expectation of pain with normal activity -Excessive focus on pain -Feeling out of control -Passivity towards rehabilitation	-Lack of sleep secondary to pain -History of other disabling injuries or conditions
Affective Factors	**Waddell's Signs**
-Poor work history -Poor Compliance with exercise -Withdrawal from activities -History of substance abuse -Depression -Irritability -Anxiety -Lack of socialization -History of Physical or Psychological abuse	-Pain with axial loading of the spine -Superficial tenderness to palpation (light touch) -Overreaction (pain out of proportion to physical findings) -Straight leg raise test improves with distraction -Regional weakness

an acute process. Be sure to instruct the patient to stand in a relaxed fashion, as patients will frequently stand in a more 'correct' fashion for inspection by the physician. A patient standing with their weight predominately on one side will clue your thinking to a possible leg-length discrepancy or a closed dysfunction on the opposite side of the lumbar spine.

After a gross inspection, one should look for any un-leveling. The shoulders, fingertips, ASIS, patella, malleoli, PSIS, and gluteal folds should be level and symmetrical to the midline. Inspection for anteroposterior & rotational/transverse plane asymmetries requires a 'walk-around' the patient – inspecting only the front or the right side of a patient may hide asymmetries for the hasty physician. Any asymmetry will clue the examiner to a possible somatic dysfunction at that level.

Look for gross deformity next. One should look for scoliosis, kyphosis or lordosis, as well as rotational/transverse plane asymmetries. One should inspect further for the presence of foot, ankle, knee, or hip abnormalities. These gross deformities can be the primary cause of low back pain or may represent a compensatory mechanism from another problem.

Gait

The observation of the gait should begin with the question of whether it appears normal or not. It is a simple task but can give a lot of information. One should be looking for limitations and asymmetry in the gait. For example, a person with an acute strain of the iliocostalis and subsequent restrictions of the SI-joint and facet joints will have a limitation in the length of the stride. When beginning your experience with gait analysis, look at the arms and legs for asymmetry of motion – their longer course during gait magnifies abnormal motions. Asking the patient to walk quickly will also give you an advantage as the patient will have less compensation time to correct for abnormal mechanics. This process takes multiple passes initially!

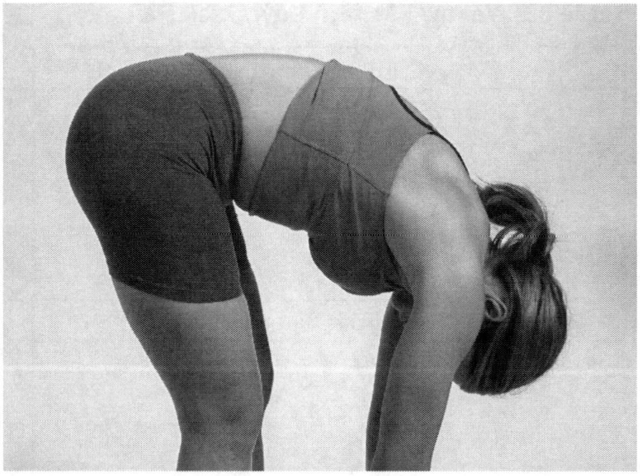

Figure 6.2. Flexion of the lumbar spine.

Range of Motion

The gross range of motion has nearly as much variability as there are personalities. Despite these vast differences in patients, knowing the normal ranges of motions will aid in identifying the source of the problem and will later help in determining response to your treatment.

The assessment of the gross motion of the lumbosacral spine is performed with the patient standing. In this assessment, it is important to assure that one is actually measuring the range of motion in the lumbar spine and not in the pelvis, knees or thoracic spine[5] and it should be measured in degrees (Table 6.3).

Table 6.3. Movements of the Lumbar Spine

Forward Flexion	(40 to 60°)
Extension	(20 to 35°)
Lateral Flexion	(15 to 20°)
Rotation	(3 to 18°)

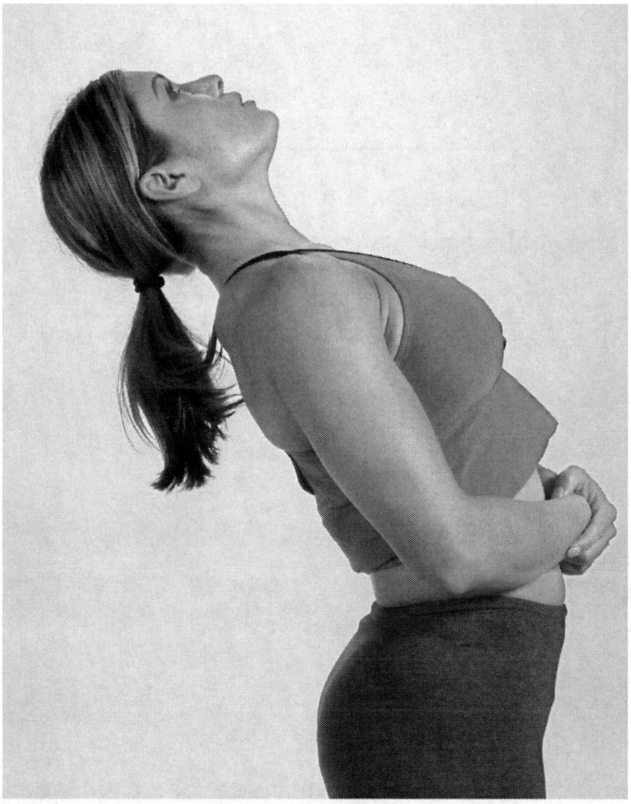

Figure 6.3. Extension of the lumbar spine.

Forward flexion of the lumbar spine is the motion that can easily be negligible but appear to be normal due to compensatory mechanisms. During lumbar flexion, the examiner should see the normal lordotic curve of the lumbar spine disappear (Figure 6.2). The examiner can further confirm true lumbar flexion by placing one thumb on the spinous process of L1 and the other on the base of the sacrum. The examiner should see thumbs separate. The same principles can be applied when assessing the other planes of motion (Figures 6.3, 6.4 and 6.5).

Segmental Motion

The assessment of the individual motion of the various segments relative to each other is one of the crucial elements in making an exact diagnosis. The history and evaluation of gross ROM will typically tell you if the dysfunction is in the lumbosacral spine but it is the examiner's challenge to find which specific dysfunctions have led this patient to your office. Before visualizing the dynamics of motion, one should understand the basics first. One must know the difference between various types of barriers (Figure 6.6). The anatomic barrier (AB) is the barrier created by the anatomy of the body. It is formed by ligaments, tendons and bones. It is the limit to passive motion.[6] The physiological barrier (PB) is the end-point at which a person can actively move. It is within the anatomical barriers. The restrictive (a.k.a., pathologic) barrier (RB) is created by the dysfunction or dysfunctions and decreases the range of motion short of the physiological barrier.[6] For example, a patient may be able to flex the lumbar spine to 30 degrees but from 20 to 30 degrees it is painful. Twenty degrees is the restrictive barrier and 30 degrees is the physiologic barrier.

Knowing the normal range of motion is important but even more important is looking for symmetry. If a patient is able to sidebend the lumbosacral spine to 20 degrees in one direction and only 10 degrees to the other, one must use this piece of information to localize the underlying cause.

Any lumbosacral examination is not fully complete without evaluation of hamstring flexibility. With its origination on the pelvis (and in a number of individuals, a portion of the tendon continues over the ischial tuberosity, blending directly with the posterior sacroiliac ligament), the hamstrings have a direct link to the pelvis and sacrum, and can possibly create dysfunctions. For example, hamstrings with decreased flexibility will create a vector force with the

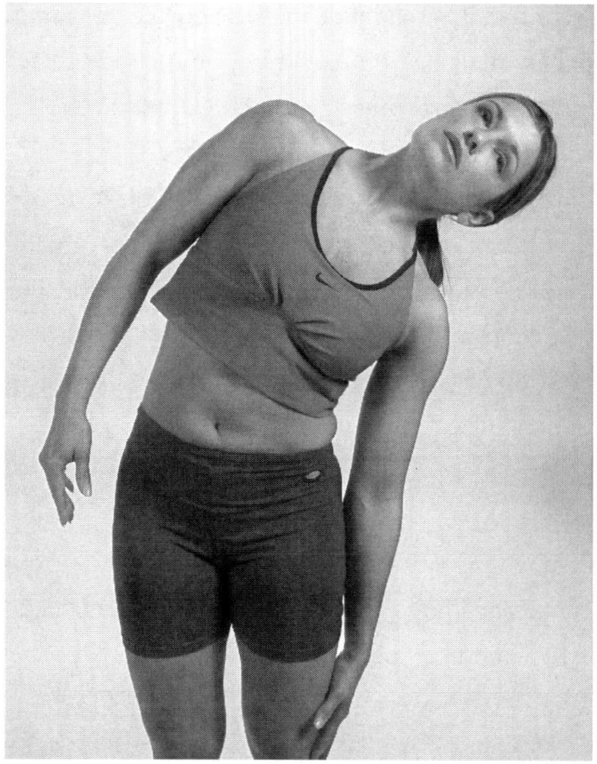

Figure 6.4. Side-bending of the lumbar spine.

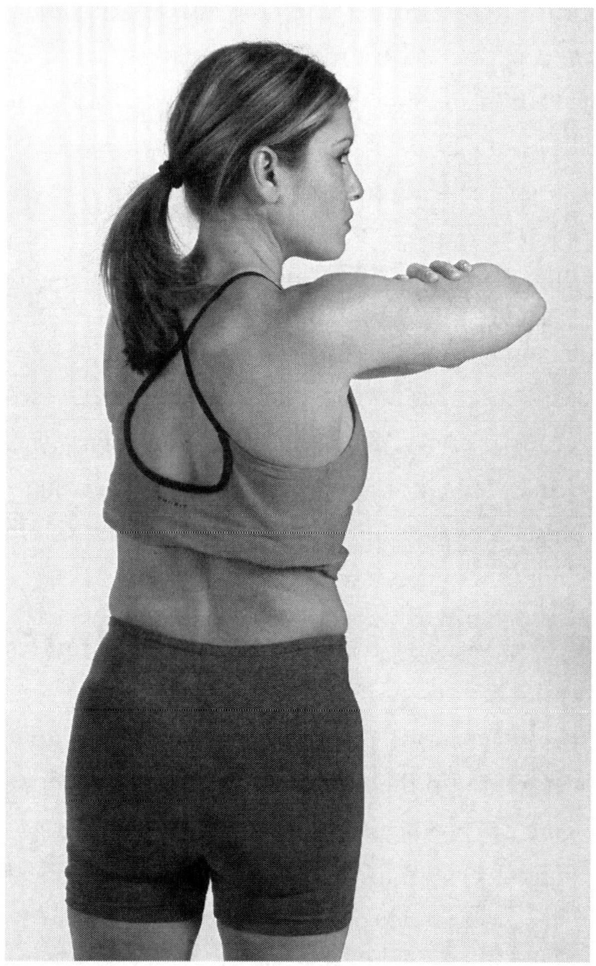

Figure 6.5. Rotation of the lumbar spine.

result being a tendency towards posterior rotation of the pelvis. This has a direct effect on the sacro-iliac joint and the lumbar musculature connected to the pelvis (quadratus lumborum, erector spinae). Assessing the hamstring flexibility is a passive test, performed by the examiner lifting the heel of the patient's leg with the knee extended, until an endpoint is reached (the opposite leg begins to lift off the exam table). Compare with the opposite leg. The normal range is 60-120 degrees, depending on the patient.

Palpation

Trained palpation is the tool that gives the osteopathic physician a huge advantage in musculoskeletal complaints. After hundreds of patients, an examiner will "get a feel" for the normal and the abnormal. Palpation is like driving a car: you can read about it and see it done, but it's not until you do it a few dozen times that it starts to feel comfortable. By palpating the lumbosacral region in every patient, one will get more proficient with each encounter. Palpation should begin by excluding non-musculoskeletal ailments, e.g., palpating for costo-vertebral angle and suprapubic tenderness will help to exclude infections of the G.U. tract. Percussion of the spinous processes will aid in excluding possible infections of the vertebrae or discitis.

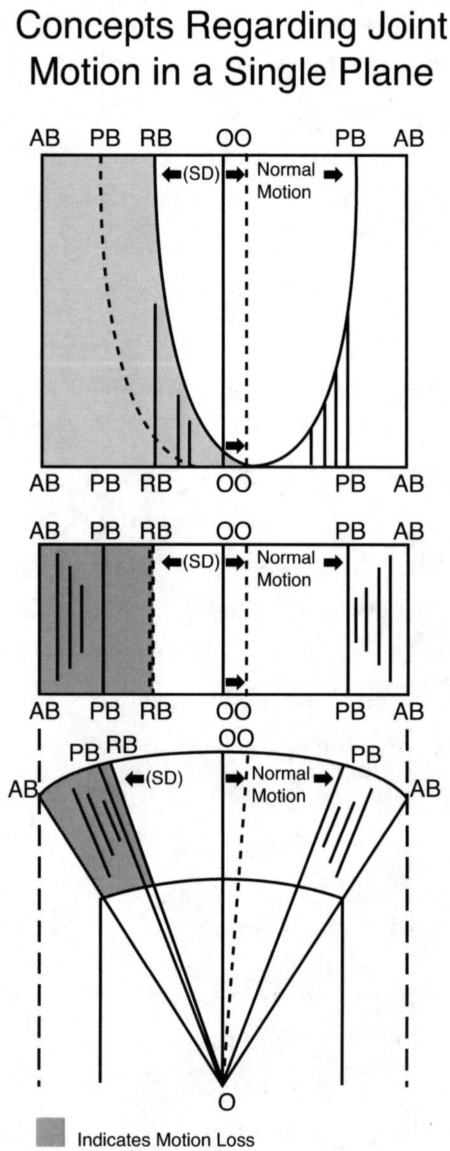

Figure 6.6. Barrier concept in somatic dysfunction.

Many osteopathic texts and medical schools use the acronym TART. The four criteria are: (T)issue texture changes, (A)symmetry of landmarks, (R)estriction of motion and (T)enderness to palpation.[6] This is a wonderfully convenient and easy to remember acronym that allows the examiner to identify somatic dysfunctions.

By first touching the tissue, one will get a feel for the turgor and tone of the tissue. The regions with increased turgor and tone commonly are the location of the dysfunctions. By palpating the dysfunctions, one can assess the severity of the strain patterns. Typically, one will find restrictions in the motion of fascia. Your palpatory findings will typically be confirming the acute or chronic process elicited in your history. Acute dysfunctions typically have a warm, boggy feel with focal tender points. The tender points in acute processes are usually sharp and severe,[7] while chronic processes have a firmer feel and diffuse tender points,[7] which are frequently described as being 'sore' instead of 'tender.'

Beneath the muscle and fascia are the lumbar vertebrae and sacrum. One should begin by pressing the transverse processes of the vertebrae anteriorly (inducing rotation) and assessing the ease of motion of right and left rotation. As described earlier, dysfunctions are named for the direction they want to go and are named in relation to the anterior body of the vertebrae. For example, if L4 rotates to the right more easily (pressing down is easier on the left transverse process) than to the right, it is described as being rotated right. By palpating the spinous processes of the individual vertebrae an examiner will be able to find spina bifida occulta (absence or irregular gap of the spinous processes) or spondylolisthesis (the spinous process and the entire lumbar vertebra seem to be much more anterior than the remaining vertebrae).

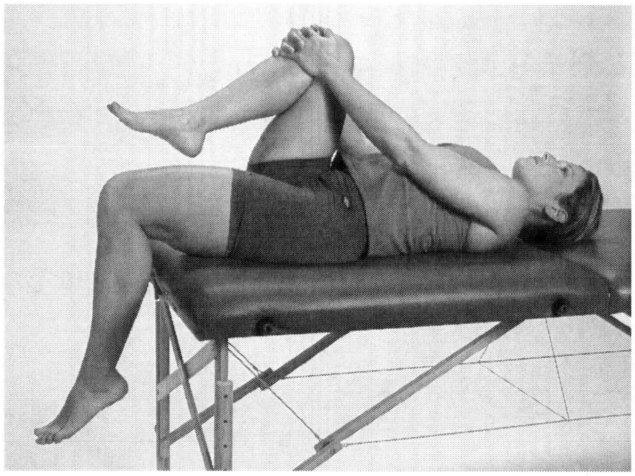

Figure 6.7. Thomas Test.

A tight iliopsoas can also be a cause of low back pain. Due to its origin from the ilium, a tight iliopsoas can create an undue force on the pelvis.

The ***Thomas Test*** (Figure 6.7) is used to assess the tone of the iliopsoas. A supine patient begins with both legs extended and then passively flexes one leg to the chest. In a positive test (the result of a tight iliopsoas on the contralateral side) the contralateral leg raises off of the table. Normally, the contralateral leg will remain flat. Compare both sides.

Neurovascular Examination

At this time in the examination, one typically has a good idea of the source of pain, the severity and the patient's limitations. Whether this is the case or one needs further confirmation, the examination is not complete without a neurological examination and certain hallmark tests. These hallmark tests are important to support your diagnosis and exclude others. The most critical test is the diagnosis of nerve root compromise.

The neurological evaluation should include Achilles (S1) and patellar (L2-4) reflex testing, ankle and great toe dorsiflexion (L4-L5) and plantarflexion (S1) strength, as well as the location of sensory complaints (dermatomes involved). Light touch testing for sensation in the medial (L4), dorsal (L5), and lateral (S1) aspects of the foot should also be performed. In patients presenting with acute LBP and no specific limb complaints, a more elaborate neurological exam is not usually necessary. A seated and supine straight leg raise test (SLR) evaluates for nerve root impingement. This abbreviated neurological evaluation of the lower extremity allows detection of clinically significant nerve root compromise at the L4-L5 or L5-S1 levels. These two sites make up over 90% of all significant radiculopathy secondary to lumbar disc herniation.

Further reflexes are evaluated via the ***Babinski*** and ***Oppenheimer's Signs.*** Both are looking for an upper motor neuron defect caused by a disc herniation and are positive if the great toe dorsiflexes.

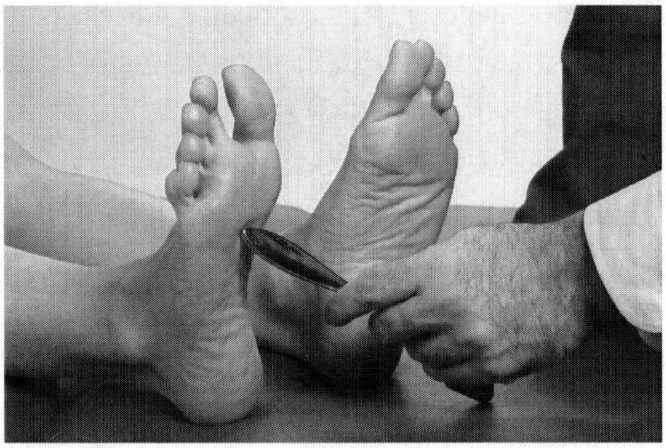

Figure 6.8. Babinski Sign.

The ***Babinski Sign*** is conducted by taking a sharp object such as a key or the handle of a reflex hammer and rubbing it along the lateral aspect of the foot and crossing over to the skin overlying the plantar surface of the metatarsophalangeal joints (Figure 6.8).

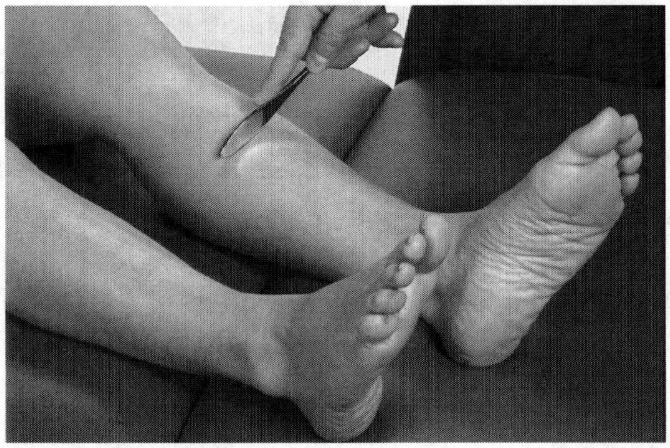

Figure 6.9. Oppenheimer's Sign.

The ***Oppenheimer's Sign*** involves taking a blunt object and sliding it down the medial aspect of the leg (Figure 6.9).

Strength testing is a brief, but invaluable, piece of information. Leg extension will evaluate L4 while dorsiflexion of the great toe and plantar flexion of the foot will evaluate L5 and S1, respectively. It may also lead you to understand the reason the pathophysiology began in the first place – e.g., weak and tight adductors leading to recurrent pubic symphysis dysfunctions – and therefore, elicitation of the true etiology.

Light touch of the medial (L4), dorsal (L5) and lateral (S1) aspects of the foot will assess the sensory portion of those nerve roots. Any asymmetry or abnormality in those regions should be considered pertinent.

PROVOCATIVE TESTS AND MANEUVERS

Of all the special tests, the Straight Leg Raise (SLR) test is one of the most commonly described and documented tests – this also means it is misinterpreted and misapplied quite often as well! A variant of this is the crossed straight leg test. Both are assessing for irritation/inflammation of the sciatic nerve root, most commonly due to lumbar disc herniation, although there are other etiologies (lumbar spondyloarthropathy, viral inflammation, femoral/acetabular arthropathy, and piriformis syndrome, to name a few).

Straight Leg Raising Test (SLR) - BASIC EXAM. With the patient lying supine, the patient relaxes his or her leg and the leg with knee extended is passively raised off the examination table by the examiner (Figure 6.10).

Positive Test: A radicular pain emanating from the low back following the sciatic nerve distribution, and usually radiating below the knee on the ipsilateral side.

Indicates: Nerve root impingement. **(NOTE: It is critical to ascertain whether the radicular pain the patient is complaining of is the pain the test provokes – some patients will have pain with orthopedic or neurological tests that have nothing to do with their pathophysiology. They may or may not have low back pain associated with this test – but if there is an absence of low back pain in a young patient, it increases the likelihood that a herniated disc is causing the problem.)**

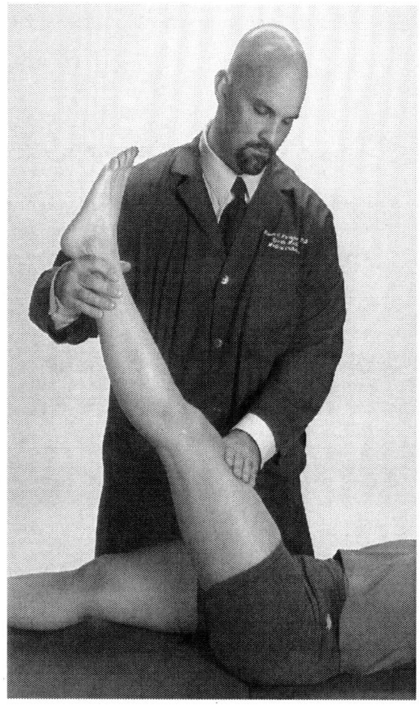

Figure 6.10. Straight Leg Raising Test.

A ***Crossed-Leg Raising Test*** is positive if pain is elicited in the opposite extremity from the one being raised.

A ***Seated Straight Leg Test - BASIC EXAM*** (Figure 6.11) is interpreted the same as the supine SLR.
One can further support nerve root entrapment by ***Bragard's Test.***[8]

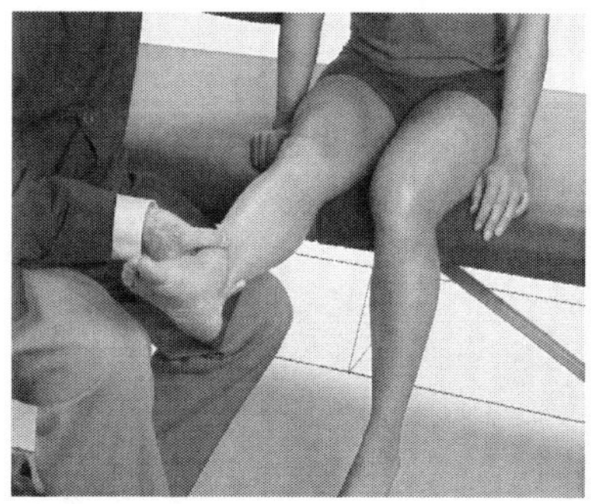

Figure 6.11. Seated Leg Raising Test.

Bragard's Test - BASIC EXAM. By taking the leg to the point just below the level of pain and adding dorsiflexion of the foot, the L5 portion of the sciatic nerve will be stretched leading to pain (Figure 6.12).

Positive Test: Pain that radiates below the knee.

Indicates: Nerve root impingement.

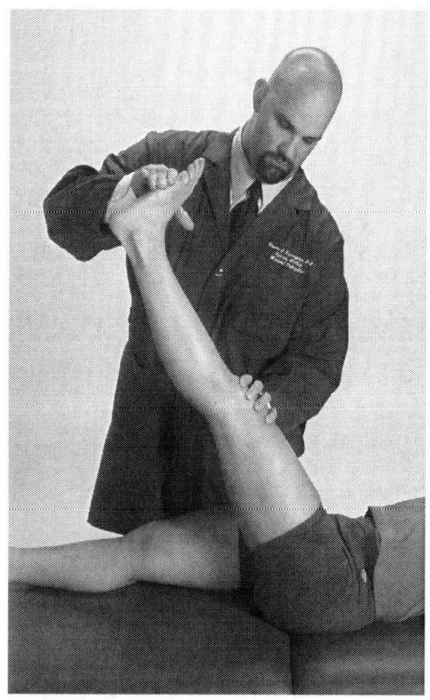

Figure 6.12. Bragard's Test.

Waddell's Sign. A common test performed in patients with possible secondary gain, this test accomplishes the same stretch of the sciatic nerve as the straight leg test but the patient is sitting on the examination table with the legs hanging over the edge, this is a Seated Straight Leg Raise.

The examiner takes the patient's leg and extends it (see Figure 6.11).

Positive Test: Pain in the back radiating below the knee.

Indicates: Nerve root impingement. However, it is a positive

Waddell's Sign if the supine SLR is positive and the seated SLR is negative.

Hoover Test. This is another test for a possible malingering patient. With the patient lying supine, the examiner places a hand under each heel. The patient is then asked to lift the affected leg off the table (Figure 6.13). A normal response is for the patient to push downward with the contralateral heel.

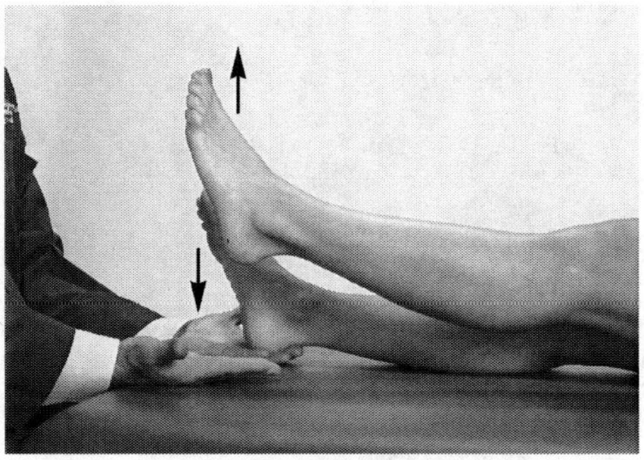

Figure 6.13. Hoover Test.

Positive Test: If no downward force is felt, the patient is not giving enough effort.

Indicates: The patient may be malingering, or seeking a secondary gain.

A test for Spondylolysis should be considered in patients who are participating in hyperextension activities and have pain on provocative tests.

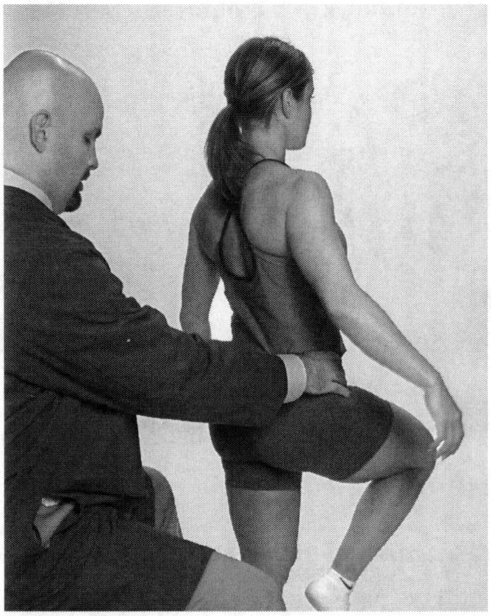

Figure 6.14a. Stork Test.

Stork Test. This is a single leg weight-bearing hyperextension test where the patient stands on one leg and then leans backward extending the lower back (Figures 6.14a and 6.14b).

Positive Test: When the patient experiences pain in the low back, as this stresses the posterior elements of the spine on the ipsilateral side.

Indicates: A possible pars defect/stress fracture, spondylolysis, or facet pathology. Remember this could be a bilateral fracture, which sets the patient up for a spondylolisthesis.

Kemp's Test - BASIC EXAM. This is performed like the ***Stork Test*** except that both feet are on the floor (or the patient is seated) and the examiner provides downward pressure on each shoulder while the patient's lower back is hyperextended. It is interpreted exactly as the ***Stork Test***.

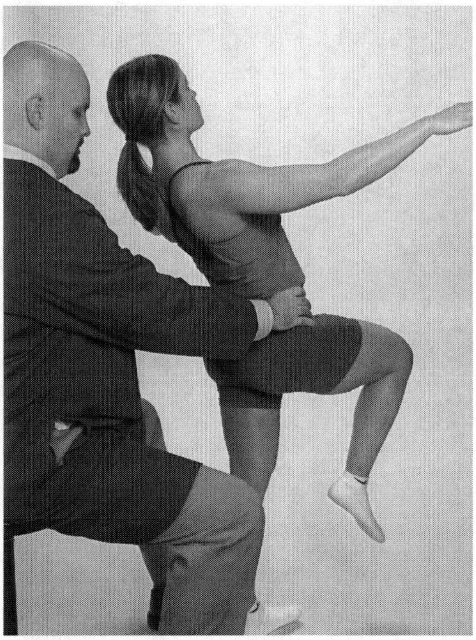

Figure 6.14b. Stork Test.

COMMON CONDITIONS

- Psoas spasm (psoas syndrome)
- Flexed non-neutral upper lumbar dysfunction
- Extended non-neutral low lumbar dysfunction
- Neutral somatic dysfunction
- Piriformis syndrome
- Leg length inequality and pelvic tilt syndrome
- Muscle imbalance of the trunk (including scoliosis) or lower extremities
- Spondylolysis/pars defects/stress fractures
- Spondylolisthesis
- Herniated/bulging disc
- Nerve root irritation (mechanical, chemical, etc.)
- Muscular strain
- Fractures (compression, spinous process, etc.)

CONDITIONS THAT SHOULD NOT BE MISSED DUE TO MORBIDITY OR MORTALITY

The Differential diagnosis for low back pain.

Table 6.4. Highlighting Conditions that Should Never be Missed

System	Conditions
Vascular	**Expanding (dissecting) Aortic aneurysm**
Gastrointestinal	**Pancreatitis** **Peptic Ulcers** Cholecystitis **Colonic Cancer**
Genitourinary	Endometriosis **Tubal Pregnancy** **Kidney Stones** Prostatitis Chronic Pelvic Inflammatory disease **Perinephric Abscess** **Pyelonephritis**
Endocrinologic/ Metabolic	Osteoporosis Osteomalacia Hyperparathyroidism **Paget's Disease** Acromegaly **Cushing's Disease** Ochronosis

Table 6.4 Continues on next page.

Table 6.4. Relationship of Discs and Exiting Nerve Roots in the Lumbar Spine (Continued)

System	Conditions
Hematologic	Hemoglobinopathy Mylofibrosis Mastocytosis
Rheumatologic	**Spondyloathropathies** **Ankylosing Spondylitis** **Reiter's Syndrome** **Psoriatic Arthritis** **Enteropathic Arthritis** **Bechet's Syndrome** Familial Mediterranean Fever Whipple's disease Diffuse Idiopathic Skeletal Hyperostosis
Psychogenic	Affective Disorder Conversion Disorder Somatization Disorder Malingering
Infection	**Osteomyelitis** **Epidural/paraspinal abscess** **Disc Space Infection** **Pyogenic Sacroiliitis**
Neoplastic	**Skeletal Metastases** **Spinal Cord Tumors** **Leukemia** **Lymphoma** **Retroperitoneal Tumors** **Primary Lumbosacral Tumors** Benign **Malignant**
Miscellaneous	**Sarcoidosis** **Subacute Endocarditis** **Retroperitoneal Fibrosis** **Herpes Zoster** **Fat Herniation of Lumbar Space** **Multiple myeloma** **Neurologic deficit with Cauda Equina Syndrome** (paralysis of lower extremities, fecal/urinary incontinence, saddle anessthesia etc.)

REFERENCES:

1. Deyo RA, Weinstein JN. Low back pain. *New England Journal of Medicine.* 2001;344: 363-370.
2. Hart LG, Deyo RA, Cherkin DC. Physician office visits for low back pain. Frequency, clinical evalulation, and treatment patterns from an U.S. national survey. *Spine,* 1995; 20: 9-11.
3. Frymoyer JW, Cats-Baril WL. An overview of the incidence and costs of low back pain. *Orthopedic Clinics of North America.* 1991; 22: 263-71.
4. Drezner JA, Herring SA. Managing low-back pain: Steps to optimize function and hasten return to activity. *The Physician and Sports Medicine.* 2001;29:(8): 37-43.
5. Magee DJ. *Orthopedic Physical Assessment.* 5th ed. Toronto: W.B. Saunders Company; 2008.
6. American Osteopathic Association. *Foundations for Osteopathic Medicine.* Philadelphia: Williams & Wilkins; 1997.
7. Kuchera WA, Kuchera ML. *Osteopathic Principles in Practice.* Revised 2nd ed. Columbus, Ohio: Greyden Press; 1992.
8. Seidel HM, Ball JW et al. *Mosby' Guide to Physical Examination.* 4th Ed. 1999; 728.
9. Atlas SJ, Deyo RA. Evaluating and managing acute low back pain in the primary care setting. Journal of *General Internal Medicine.* 2001;16:120-131.
10. Balague F, Mannion AF, Pellise F, Cedraschi C. Clinical update: Low back pain. *Lancet.* 2007;369:726-8.
11. Bigos S, Bowyer O, Braen G et al. Acute low back problems in adults. Clinical Practice Guideline. No.14. AHCPR publication No. 95-0642.
12. Chou R, Qaseem A, Snow V et al. Diagnosis and treatment of low back pain: A joint practice guideline from the American College of Physicians and the American Pain Society. *Ann Intern Med.* 2007;147:478-91.
13. Kinkade S. Evaluation and treatment of acute low back pain. *Am Fam Physician.* 2007;75:1181-8.
14. Kovacs FM, Abraira V, Zamora J et al. Correlation between pain, disability, and quality of life in patients with common low back pain. I. 2004;29:206-210.
15. Manek NJ, MacGregor AJ. Epidemiology of back disorders: Prevalence, risk factors, and prognosis. *Current Opinion in Rheumatology.* 2005;17:134-140.
16. Reis S, Borkan J, Van Raalte R et al. The LBP patient perception scale: A new predictor of LBP episode outcomes among primary care patients. *Patient Educ Couns.* 2007;67:191-5.
17. Rives PA, Douglass AB. Evaluation and treatment of low back pain in family practice. *J Am Board Fam Pract.* 2004;17 (suppl):S23-31.

7 The Hip Exam

John J. Dougherty, D.O., FAOASM

ANATOMY

The term "hip" has a broad common definition traditionally including the acetabular-femoral joint, pelvis and sacroiliac spine. For this discussion the "hip" joint will be defined as the acetabular-femoral joint.

The hip is classified as a ball and socket joint and has a unique set of factors contributing to its stability and function. Factors affecting the biomechanical integrity of the joint include muscular attachments, cartilaginous and ligamentous structures, as well as the joints above and below the central hub. Alteration of the relationship between the femur and acetabular fossa can result in undue wear and eventual disruption of the cartilaginous surfaces within the joint and therefore, pain.

Medially, superior, and posterior, the hip is loaded via the sacroiliac joint, which transmits weight from the axial spine. Located medial, anterior, and inferior, the pubic symphysis functions as a point of stabilization, doing so for both hips. These points of attachment can affect the angle and rotation of the acetabular fossa. Inferiorly, the stability and alignment of the lower extremities kinetic chain can affect the seating of the femoral head into the acetabular fossa.

A fibrous capsule encases the acetabular-femoral joint forming the central joint cavity. It originates at the acetabular rim and inserts on the intertrochanteric line of the femur and its neck posteriorly. This capsule is lined by a synovial layer that secretes the viscous synovial fluid. The iliofemoral ligament is a Y-shaped band anterior to the capsule that in consort with the posterior ischiofemoral ligament prevents hyperextension. The joint is additionally reinforced anteriorly and inferiorly with the pubofemoral ligament with the duty of resisting over abduction when in extension and abduction. The ligamentum teres anchors the head of the femur to the acetabulum inferior and anterior and carries a small artery to the head of the femur. The acetabular fossa is covered with hyaline cartilage, as is the femoral head. A meniscal like fibro-cartilaginous labrum rims and therefore, deepens the fossa. This extension allows for load redistribution as the joint experiences weight transfer.

Muscular support of the hip is best described by function. Flexion and extension are the primary movements of the joint. The Iliopsoas serves as the primary flexor with the rectus femoris, adductor group and the other muscles passing anterior to the pelvic rim being secondary flexors. Extension is accomplished primarily by the gluteus maximus in collaboration with the medial and lateral hamstring complexes. These muscle groups act as restraint to the opposing contracting group.

Rotation of the joint is not as full as that seen in the shoulder, but still a crucial function. The rotator cuff of the hip consists of primarily two groups of muscles: the abductors and external rotators. The gluteus medius acts as the primary abductor with secondary contribution from the gluteus minimus. Insertion for both is into the anterior, lateral aspect of the greater trochanter in the peripheral compartment pulling toward their origin at the posterior rim of the iliac crest. External rotators attaching at the posterior lateral aspect of the greater trochanter include the piriformis, superior and inferior gemelius, obturator internus and externus, and the quadratus femoris.

Table 7.1. Muscles of the Hip Joint

Muscle	Origin	Insertion	Innervation	Nerve Root
Flexion				
Iliopsoas Psoas Minor	Sides of T12-L1 vertebrae	Pectineal line, iliopectineal eminence of femur	Ventral rami of lumbars	L1, L2
Psoas Major	Sides of the T12 – L5 vertebrae	Lesser trochanter of femur	Ventral rami of lumbars	L1, L2, L3
Iliacus	Iliac crest, iliac fossa, ala of sacrum, anterior sacroiliac ligaments	Lesser trochanter and femur distal to, tendon of psoas major	Femoral	L2, L3
Sartorius	Anterior superior iliac spine (ASIS)	Superior medial tibia	Femoral	L2, L3
Pectineus	Superior ramus of pubis	Pectineal line, just inferior to lesser trochanter	Femoral	L2, L3
Rectus femoris	ASIS and ilium superior to acetabulum	Base of patella, patellar ligamant	Femoral	L2, L3, L4
Adductor brevis	Body and inferior pubic ramus	Pectineal line, proximal linea aspera	Obturator	L2, L4
Adductor magnus	Inferior pubic ramus, ischial ramus	Gluteal tuberosity, linea aspera, medial supracondylar line	Obturator	L2-L4
Adductor longus	Body and inferior pubic ramus	Middle 1/3 of Linea aspera	Obturator	L2-L4
Tensor of fascia lata	Anterior Superior Iliac Spine (ASIS), Anterior Iliac crest	Iliotibial band and Gerdy's tubercle	Superior Gluteal	L5, S1
Extension				
Biceps femoris Long Head	Ischial tuberosity	Lateral fibular head, lateral collateral ligament	Tibial division of sciatic	L5, S1, S2
Biceps femoris Short Head	Linca aspera, lateral supracondylar line of femur	Lateral fibular head, lateral collateral ligament	Common fibular division of sciatic	L5, S1, S2
Semitendinosis	Ischial tuberosity	Medial superior tibial shaft	Sciatic	L5, S1, S2

Table 7.1. Muscles of the Hip Joint (Continued)

Muscle	Origin	Insertion	Innervation	Nerve Root
		Adductors		
Gracilis	Body and inferior ramus of the pubis	Superior medial tibia	Obturator	L2, L3
Pectineus	Superior ramus of pubis	Pectineal line, just inferior to lesser trochanter	Femoral	L2, L3
Adductor longus	Body and inferior pubic ramus	Middle 1/3 of Linea aspera	Obturator	L2-L4
Adductor brevis	Body and inferior pubic ramus	Pectineal line, proximal linea aspera	Obturator	L2-L4
Adductor magnus	Inferior pubic ramus, ischial ramus	Gluteal tuberosity, linea aspera, medial supracondylar line	Obturator	L2-L4
		Abductors		
Sartorius	Anterior superior iliac spine (ASIS)	Superior medial tibia	Femoral	L2, L3
Tensor fascia lata	Anterior Superior Iliac Spine (ASIS), Anterior Iliac crest	Iliotibial band and Gerdy's tubercle	Superior Gluteal	L5, S1
Obturator internus	Obturator membrane and surrounding bones	Medial aspect of greater trochanter	N. to obturator	L5, S1
Superior gemelius	Superior ischial spine, Inferior Ischia tuberosity	Medial aspect of greater trochanter	N. to obturator	L5, S1
Gluteus medius	External Ilium	Lateral Greater Trochanter	Superior Gluteal	L5, S1
Gluteus minimus	External Ilium	Anterior Greater Trochanter	Superior Gluteal	L5, S1
Gluteus maximus	Posterior Iliac wing, dorsal sacrum and coccyx	Iliotibial tract, gluteal tuberosity	Inferior Gluteal	L5, S1, S2
Piriformis	Anterior Sacrum, sacrotuberous ligament	Superior aspect of greater trochanter	Anterior Branch S1-S2	S1, S2
		External Rotators		
Sartorius	Anterior superior iliac spine (ASIS)	Superior medial tibia	Femoral	L2, L3
Obturator externus	Obturator membrane and surrounding bones	Medial aspect of greater trochanter	N. to quadratus	L3, L4

Table 7.1. Muscles of the Hip Joint (Continued)

Muscle	Origin	Insertion	Innervation	Nerve Root
External Rotators				
Obturator internus	Obturator membrane and surrounding bones	Medial aspect of greater trochanter	N. to obturator	L5, S1
Superior gemelius	Superior ischial spine, Inferior Ischial tuberosity	Medial aspect of greater trochanter	N. to obturator	L5, S1
Inferior gemelius	Superior ischial spine, Inferior Ischial tuberosity	Medial aspect of greater trochanter	N. to quadratus	L5, S1
Quadratus femoris	Lateral border of ischial tuberosity	Quadrate tubercle of femur	N. to quadratus	L5, S1
Gluteus medius	External Ilium	Lateral Greater Trochanter	Superior Gluteal	L5, S1
Gluteus maximus	Posterior Iliac wing, dorsal sacrum and coccyx	Iliotibial tract, gluteal tuberosity	Inferior Gluteal	L5, S1, S2
Piriformis	Anterior Sacrum, sacrotuberous ligament	Superior aspect of greater trochanter	Anterior Branch S1-S2	S1, S2
Internal Rotators				
Iliopsoas Psoas Minor	Sides of T12-L1 vertebrae	Pectineal line, iliopectineal eminence of femur	Ventral rami of lumbars	L1,L2
Psoas Major	Sides of the T12 – L5 vertebrae	Lesser trochanter of femur	Ventral rami of lumbars	L1,L2,L3
Iliacus	Iliac crest, iliac fossa, ala of sacrum, anterior sacroiliac ligaments	Lesser trochanter and femur distal to, tendon of psoas major	Femoral	L2,L3
Pectineus	Superior ramus of pubis	Pectineal line, just inferior to lesser trochanter	Femoral	L2, L3
Gracilis	Body and inferior ramus of the pubis	Superior medial tibia	Obturator	L2, L3
Tensor fascia lata	Anterior Superior Iliac Spine (ASIS), Anterior Iliac crest	Iliotibial band and Gerdy's tubercle	Superior Gluteal	L5, S1
Gluteus Medius -anterior fibers	External Ilium	Lateral Greater Trochanter	Superior Gluteal	L5, S1
Gluteus minimus - anterior fibers	External Ilium	Anterior Greater Trochanter	Superior Gluteal	L5, S1

Pelvic stabilization is maintained by the lateral and medial muscles of the hip. Medially, this is accomplished by the three adductors (longus, brevis and magnus) along with the gracilis and the pectinius. Internal rotation of the hip is a weak movement accomplished by muscles passing anterior to the joint. These include the iliopsoas and the anterior fibers of the gluteus medius and minimus.

The trochanteric region contains 3 bursae lying beneath the iliotibial band and along the greater trochanter. The largest bursa is roughly 2-4 cm in width and 4-6 cm in length and lies between the gluteus maximus tendon, the converging fibers of the tensor fascia lata where the iliotibial band is formed, and the underlying gluteus medius tendon.[1,2] The middle bursa lies between the tendons of the gluteus medius and gluteus minimus and the lateral superior border of the greater trochanter. The smallest bursa lies between the gluteus minimus and greater trochanter.[1,3] A small bursa lies below the iliopsoas tendon forming its own compartment. The purpose of these bursae is to facilitate gliding between adjacent structures.

The joint's blood supply is provided by branches of the medial and lateral femoral circumflex arteries, the artery of the femoral head, and a branch off of the obturator artery. Innervation of the region surrounding the greater trochanter is supplied by branches of the iliohypogastric nerve, the obturator, femoral and sciatic nerves, as well as the subcostal nerve or the 2nd, 3rd, or 4th lumbar plexus.[4,8]

PHYSICAL EXAMINATION

Physical examination, as always, begins with a thorough history. The answers to the directed inquiry will lead the examiner to stratify the anticipated provocative tests/maneuvers to be inclusive or exclusive in the evaluation process.

Pain involving the hip joint can be primary or referred, and is often misdiagnosed due to common pain patterns shared with other musculoskeletal conditions. Pathology within and around the hip joint falls into one of several categories: The first is the acute onset of pain associated with trauma. Acute pain and injury has also been observed after a twisting motion. Another pathologic category can result from overuse and repetitive motion activities. The final category is diseases or degenerative conditions that may result in biomechanical alteration of the structural components of the joint.

Pain is a common clinical presentation, described as deep aching/stiffness in the hip that is occasionally sharp. Pain can be localized to the proximal, lateral aspect of the thigh and pelvic rim. Patients will often describe the pain's location by cupping their hand over the greater trochanteric region. The pain may radiate into the groin and at times down the lateral aspect of the thigh.[4,5] Pain can be confused with pain referred from the lumbosacral spine or sciatic nerve.[4,6] At times, a catching or locking of the joint is noted. The pain can be referred to the level of the knee and is rarely found to be more distal.[1] Patients may also relate numbness and symptoms in the upper thigh which do not follow a typical lumbar dermatome segment.[1]

Table 7.2. Actions of the Hip Muscles

Muscle Groups	Function: as it relates to the Hip Joint					
Anterior/Medial	**Flexion**	**Extension**	**Adduction**	**Abduction**	**External Rotation**	**Internal Rotation**
Psoas Minor	X					when flexed
Psoas Major	X					when flexed
Illiacus	X					when flexed
Gracilis			X			when flexed
Sartorius	X			X	X	
Pectineus	X	weakly	X			secondary
Rectus Femoris	X					
Adductor Brevis		weakly	X			
Adductor Magnus	X	weakly	X			
Adductor Longus		weakly	X			
Lateral						
Obturator Externus					X	
Obturator Internus				when flexed	X	
Superior Gemelli				when flexed	X	
Inferior Gemelli				when flexed	X	
Quadratus Femoris					X	
Tensor Fascia lata	X			X		anterior fibers
Gluteus Medius				X	X	anterior fibers
Gluteus Minimus				X		anterior fibers
Gluteus Maximus		X		X	X	
Piriformis				when flexed	X	
Posterior						
Biceps Femoris - Long		X				
Biceps Femoris - Short		X				
Semitendinosis		X				
Semimembranosus		X				

Pain can be made worse in the trochanteric and gluteal region by almost any movement and/or with lying on the affected side. Rising from a seated position exacerbates the condition and in certain instances patients may require a cane for ambulation. The patient may have an altered gait due to weakness from the underlying pathology or from guarding. The pain often improves with rest and gradually increases as the day progresses. Compensatory spasm in the surrounding musculature can further mask the hip pathology with overlapping pain patterns.

A history of an associated injury or fall can be insightful as to the nature of the injury itself. A past history of congenital or childhood abnormalities can be a contributing cause due to the associated altered biomechanics. When performing the physical examination of the hip, always examine the pelvis, lumbosacral spine and knee.

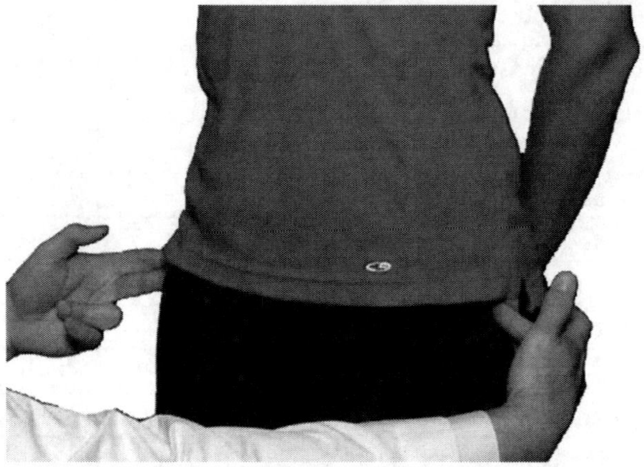

Figure 7.1. Assessment of greater trochanter asymmetry.

Observation

First observe the patient's gait for a Trendelenburg gait or employment of an assistive device. They may sit or stand in a position that relaxes the abductors and/or external rotators finding improvement of their pain in this position. Rising from a chair can induce pain with observable weakness in the affected limb by noting use of the ipsilateral upper extremity to push up from sitting.

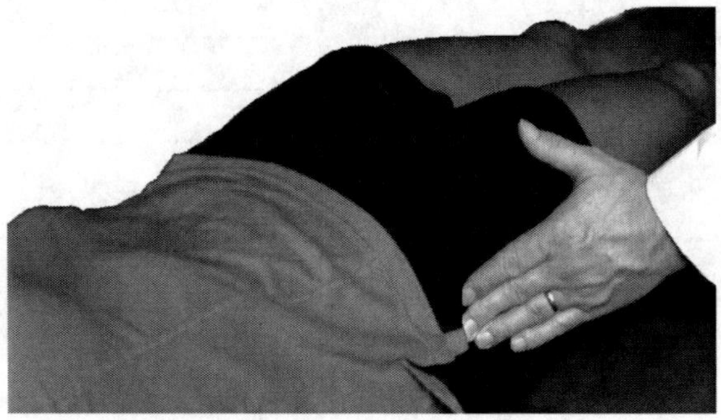

Figure 7.2. Palpation of the greater trochanter.

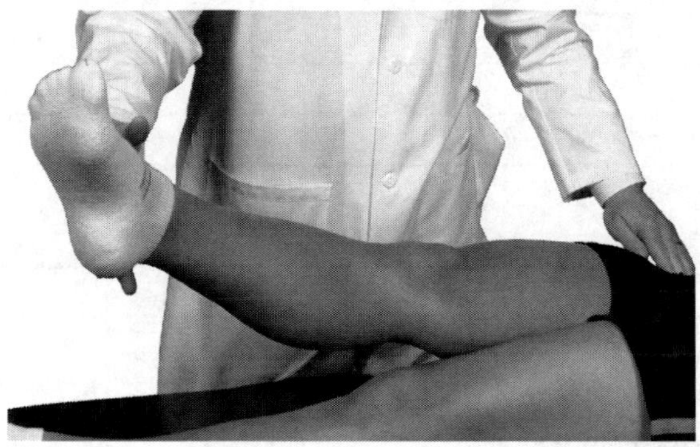

Figure 7.3. Palpation of hip flexors.

Anterior visualization includes assessment for femoral anteversion by asymmetrical prominence of the greater trochanter (Figure 7.1). A subsequent compensatory rotation of the anterior thigh can be observed. The patient may stand with weight shifted to the non-affected extremity unloading the pathologic joint. Lower extremity kinetic chain abnormalities can alter the femoral head seating and should be noted. A lateral assessment should demonstrate anatomic placement, with normal pelvic dynamics, into the acetabular fossa. Pelvic tilt, accentuated by excessive lumbar lordosis and a weakened anterior abdominal core, may result in an observable misalignment of this relationship. The superior aspect of the femoral insertion may be seated slightly counter clockwise placing the supportive ligamentous structures under additional tension. Posterior assessment identifies the presence and symmetry of gluteal folds and possible atrophy of the gluteus muscles.

Palpation

The innominate, or hip bone, is palpated with its three fused subsets in mind as each contribute different functional responsibilities. The points of attachment of the superior ilium are palpated anterior to posterior. Evaluate for abnormalities first at the Anterior Superior Iliac Spines, over the iliac crest, the external lip of the crest and finishing on the Posterior Superior Iliac Spines. The ischium is the posterior, inferior aspect of the innominate and attention is then given to palpating the prominent ischial tuberosity where an avulsion of the hamstring tendon may occur. Finishing up anterior and inferior, palpate the crest and inferior ramus of the pubis, the origin of the adductor group, identifying the femoral triangle and it's components. Within the shallow depression of the triangle lies, from medial to lateral, the femoral vein, artery and nerve (V.A.N.).

Move to palpating just below the greater trochanter, from inferior to superior. Pain causing the patient to "jump" on direct palpation inferior to and at the level of the firm bony trochanter, is referred to as "jump" sign (Figure 7.2).[3,7,8] This is indicative of lateral compartment pathology. Pain on palpation at the anterior, lateral aspect of the greater trochanter would point towards a potential pathology of the Gluteus medius or minimus at their insertion. Tenderness anterior at the iliopectinic line over the lesser trochanter may be from iliopsoas bursitis and point towards a potential hip flexor pathology (Figure 7.3). The patient may complain of a snapping sound along with this tenderness. Pain or tenderness over the SI or piriformis may be the result of compensatory problems and represent their own contibuting pathology making the underlying primary injury difficult to identify.

Range of Motion

Range of motion should be documented on all exams, preferably by goniometric measurement. Restrictions may be the result of osseous impingement, acute and/or chronic muscular spasm, ligamentous adaptation, or any combination of these.

The resting position of the hip occurs at 30° of flexion, 30° of abduction and slight external rotation. Normal range of motion is as follows:

Flexion (Figure 7.4)
120 – 135°
Extension (Figure 7.5)
15 – 30°

Abduction		Adduction	
Flexion (Horizontal) (Figure 7.6)	Knee In Extension (Figure 7.7)	Flexion (Horizontal) (Figure 7.8)	Knee In Extension (Figure 7.9)
30 – 50°	45°	60 – 70°	20 – 30°

Internal Rotation (Figure 7.10)	External Rotation (Figure 7.11)
30 – 40°	40 – 60°

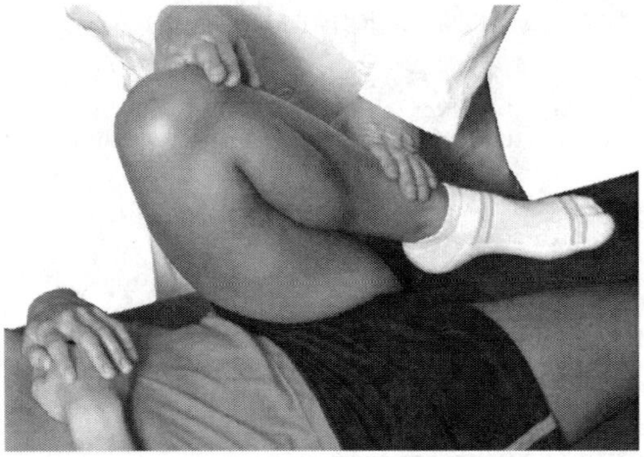

Figure 7.4. Hip flexion.

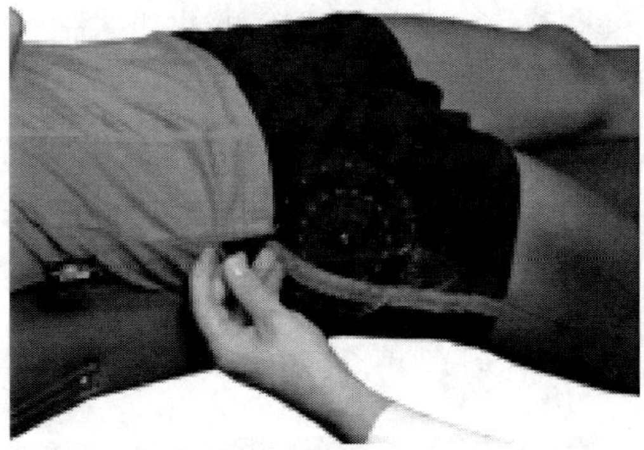

Figure 7.5. Hip extension.

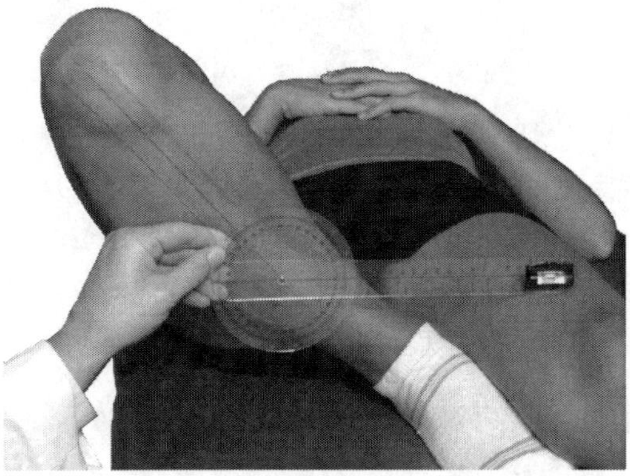

Figure 7.6. Abduction flexion.

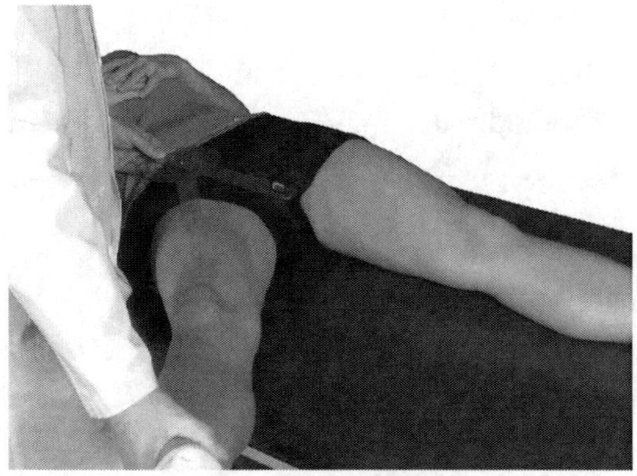

Figure 7.7. Abduction extension.

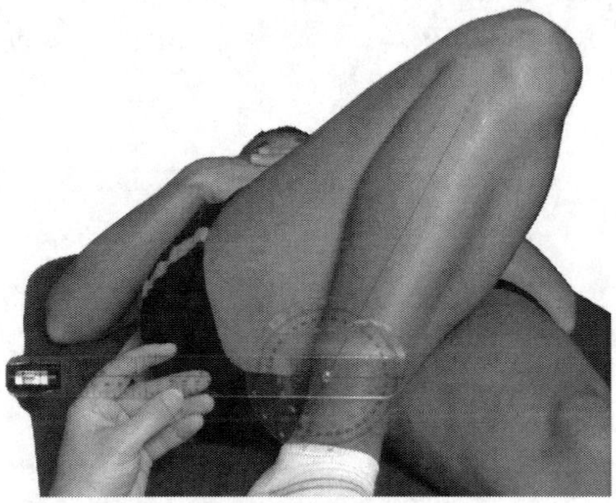

Figure 7.8. Adduction flexion.

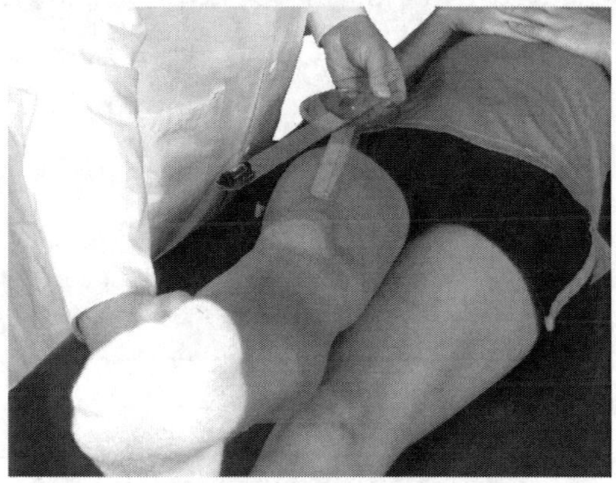

Figure 7.9. Adduction extension.

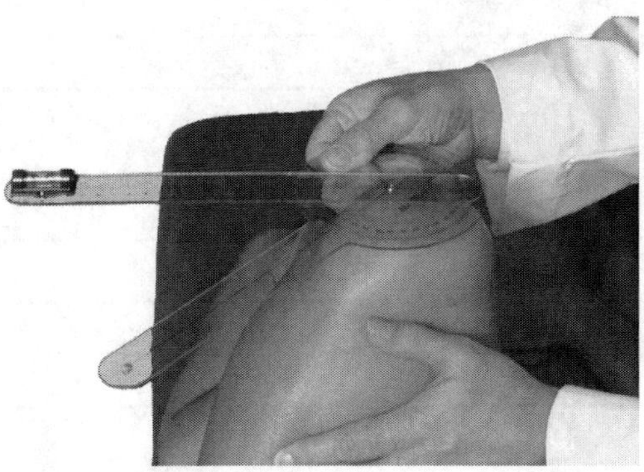

Figure 7.10. Internal rotation.

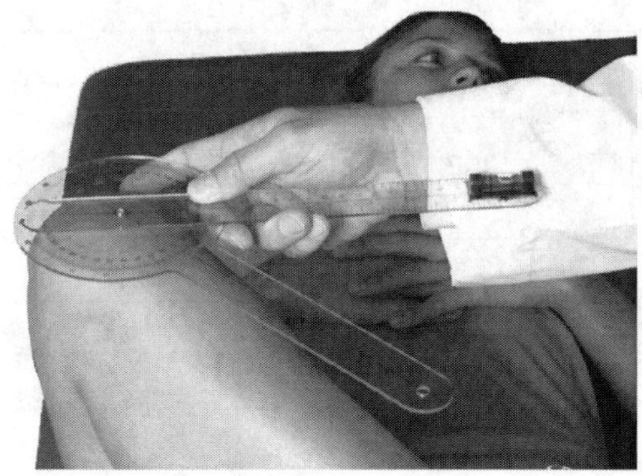

Figure 7.11. External rotation.

Neurovascular Examination

Sensory: Evaluation is undertaken by dermatomal assessment (Table 7.3).

Reflexes: Patellar (L2-L4) and Achilles (L3-L4) reflexes can assist in assessment of nerve root pathologies.

Pulses: Femoral posterior tibial and dorsalis pedis pulses should be palpated bilaterally to assess possible vascular etiology of hip pain (e.g., claudication).

Table 7.3. Dermatomes Related to the Hip

Nerve root	Dermatome
Anterior	
L1	Groin and suprapubic region
L2	Anterior thigh
L3	Lower anterior thigh and knee
L4, L5	Lower leg
Posterior	
S2-S4	Perianal

PROVOCATIVE TESTS AND MANUEVERS

Structuring the examination of the hip by a compartmental approach is presented. Manual and specific muscle testing is incorporated into this format. Beginning centrally and working out from the acetabular-femoral joint organizes the examination.

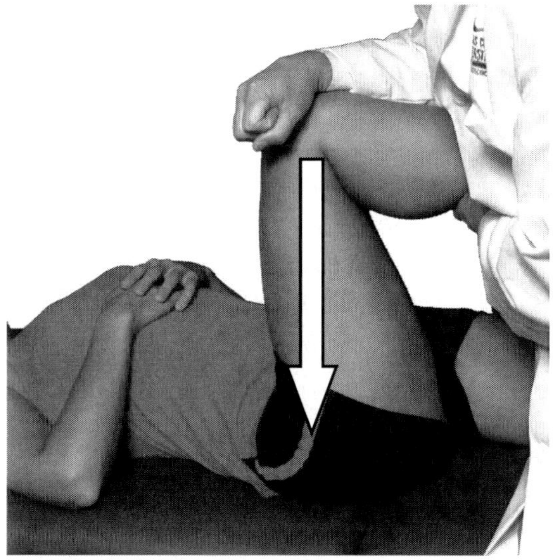

Figure 7.12. Labral loading.

Log Roll. A nonspecific exam of the hip joint performed with the patient supine. Position the affected leg on the side of the examiner. The knee is held in extension by the examiner and the foot is internally and externally rotated .

> *Positive Test*: Pain with motion. A negative evaluation does not preclude hip pathology.
>
> *Indicates*: May be nonspecific or more ominously could represent fracture of the hip.

Central Compartment Testing

Evaluation of the central compartment is performed with the integrity of the central structures in mind.

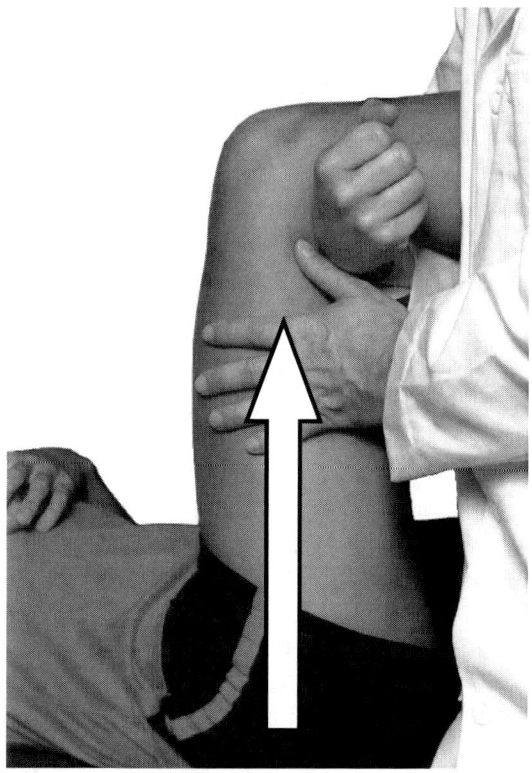

Figure 7.13. Labral distraction.

Labral Loading. Performed with the patient supine and the affected leg flexed to 90°. The examiner places the knee in the armpit compressing the femoral head into the acetabulum (Figure 7.12).

Positive Test: Pain is elicited in the hip or low back.

Indicates: A positive test points towards labral, or cartilaginous pathology.

Labral Distraction. Performed supine with hip flexed to 90°, arm under knee distracting hip up off exam table (Figure 7.13).

Positive Test: Relief of the pain from loading is considered confirmatory.

Indicates: A positive test points towards labral, or cartilaginous pathology.

Scour Test. Performed supine with hip flexed, external rotated, load into socket and articulate through annular range of motion (Figure 7.14).

Positive Test: Pain.

Indicates: Labral or articular cartilage pathology.

Apprehension Test. Performed supine with hip flexed, gently abducted and externally rotated (FABER) (Figure 7.15).

Positive Test: Anterior subluxation of the hip or anterior pain and apprehension with the FABER position. (Posterior subluxation or posterior pain and apprehension with adduction and internal rotation, indicating posterior labral pathology.)

Indicates: Anterior labral pathology. May also be positive with central hip impingement such as "CAM" or "Pincer" impingement.

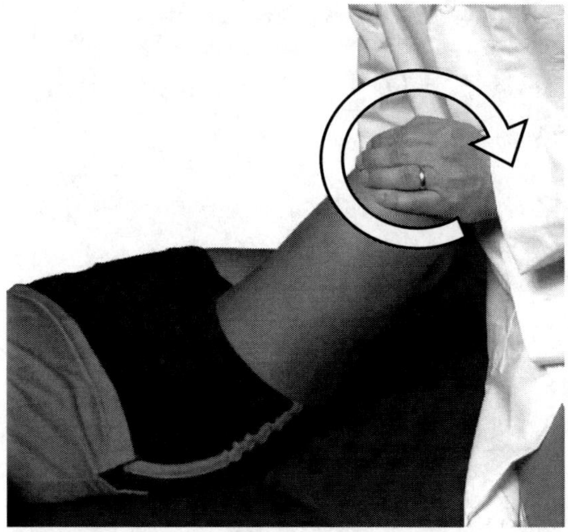

Figure 7.14. Scour Test.

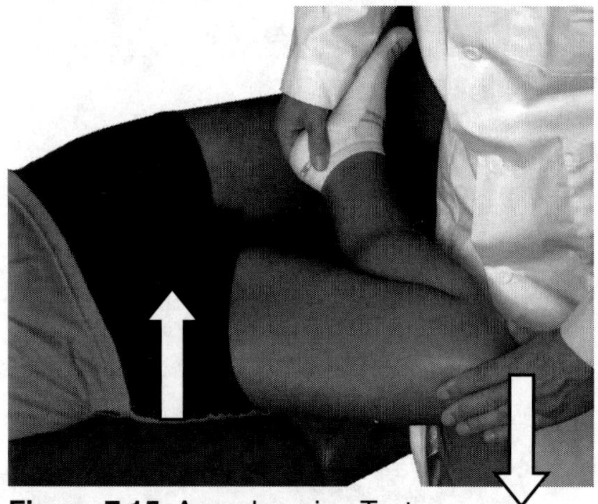

Figure 7.15. Apprehension Test.

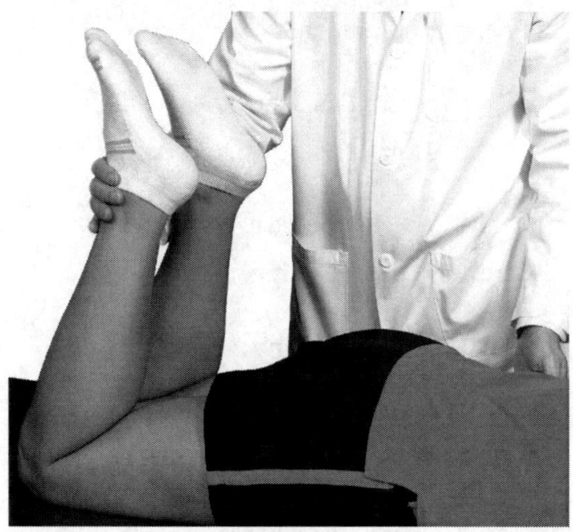

Figure 7.16. Ely's Test.

Peripheral Compartment Testing

Peripheral compartment pathology and diagnosis is primarily based on clinical symptoms.

History of catching or locking of the joint may indicate osteochromatosis (joint mouse) due to disrupted articular cartilage.

Ely's Test. Assesses the rectus femoris as it inserts on the ilium superior to acetabulum, which is part of this compartment. With the patient prone, passively flex the knees (Figure 7.16).

Positive Test: Ipsilateral hip raises off the table.

Indicates: Contracture of the rectus femoris.

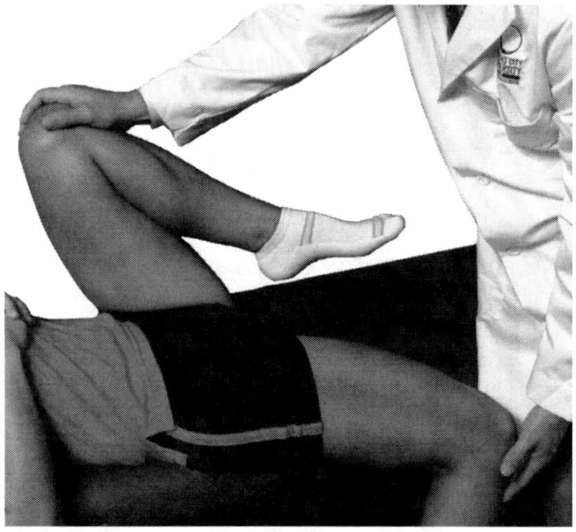

Figure 7.17. Rectus Femoris Test.

Rectus Femoris Test. Performed supine with knee bent over the edge of the table, opposite leg is brought to the chest (Figure 7.17).

Positive Test: Knee flexion to less than90°(knee off the table) while thigh flat on table.

Indicates: Rectus Femoris contraction ipsilaterally.

Lateral Compartment Testing

Straight Leg Raise Test - BASIC EXAM. Raise is performed with the patient supine. With knee in full extension lift the extremity up by the heel (Figure 7.18).

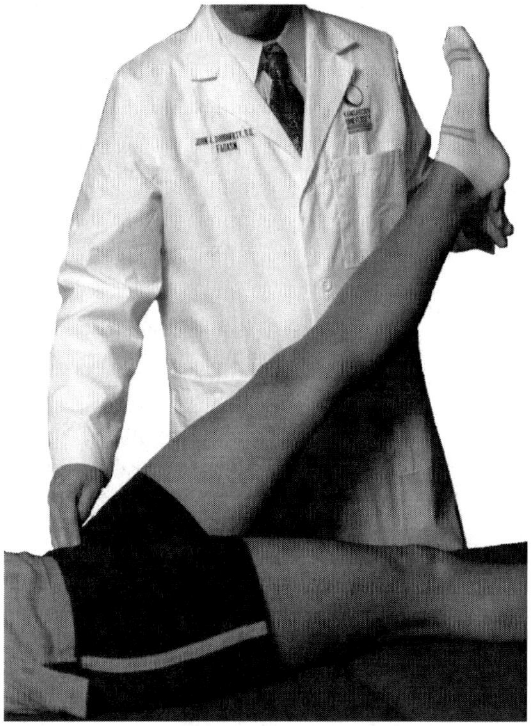

Figure 7.18. Straight Leg Raise Test.

Positive Test: Radicular pain in the first 15°-30° points towards lumbar disc etiology, or local (lateral) hip pain beyond 15° (iliotibial band slides past the trochanter).

Indicates: Lateral compartment pathology beyond 15°.

Ober's Test - BASIC EXAM. Have the patient lie on his or her side with the hips and knees flexed. The upper leg is passively abducted and extended. The limb is then lowered to the table. The hip is stabilized to prohibit the patient from rolling backward and allowing the ITB to slip over the greater trochanter (Figure 7.19).

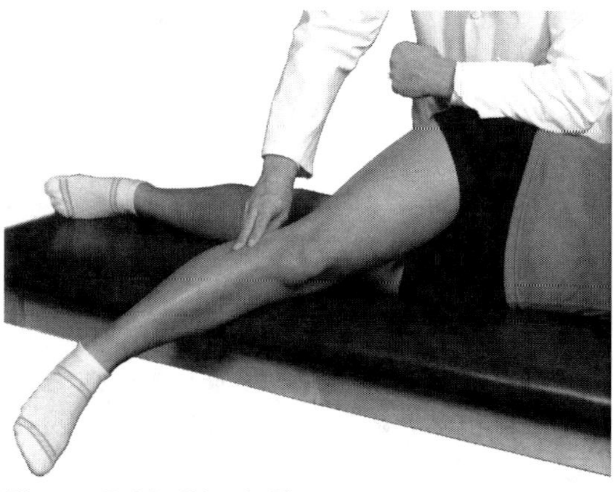

Figure 7.19. Ober's Test.

Positive Test: The leg will not fall to the table.

Indicates: Iliotibial band (ITB) contracture.

Piriformis Test. While patient lies supine, with flexed hip and knee, active hip abduction against examiner's resistance (Figure 7.20).

Positive Test: Pain over posterior aspect of the greater trochanter.

Indicates: Pirformis spasm or pathology.

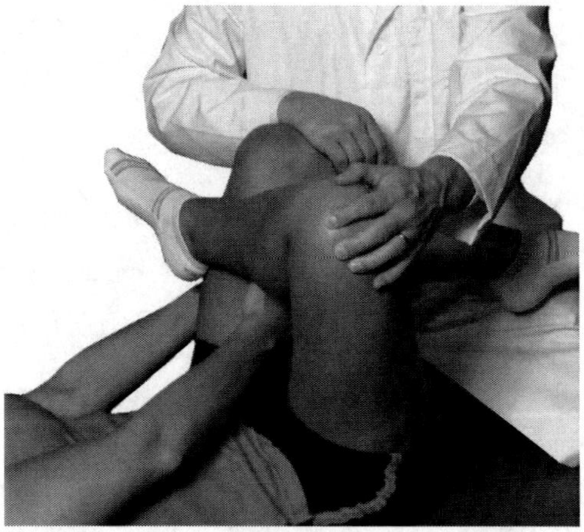

Figure 7.20. Piriformis Test.

Patrick's (FABER) Test - BASIC EXAM. Performed supine with hip flexed, gently abducted and internally rotated (Figure 7.21). The examiner then pushes the knee toward the table to further stress the hip and SI joint.

Positive Test: Pain elicited in hip joint or posteriorly near S-I.

Indicates: Hip joint pathology or S-I dysfunction depending on location of the pain.

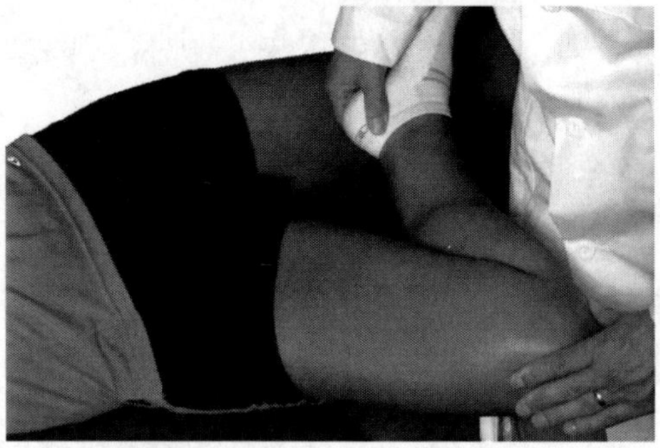

Figure 7.21. Patrick's Test.

Patrick's Test - Variation One. Place hand on lateral aspect of knee, brace contralateral ASIS and have patient externally rotate against resistance.

Positive Test: Pain or weakness in hip joint.

Indicates: May represent Gluteus medius insufficiency or pathology.

Trendelenburg's Test - BASIC EXAM. The patient stands first on one leg on the unaffected side (Figure 7.22), then the affected side, while observing for a continued level pelvis .

Positive Test: When the pelvis on the opposite side drops (Figure 7.23).

Indicates: Inability of the hip abductors to stabilize the pelvis on the femur indicates a weak or painful gluteus medius on the weight-bearing leg.

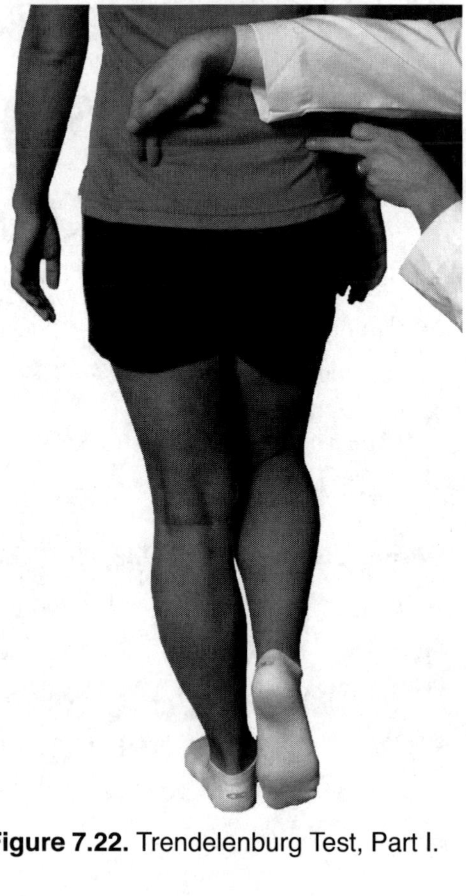

Figure 7.22. Trendelenburg Test, Part I.

Iliopsoas/Anterior Compartment Testing

There are several tests that can elicit a positive finding if the etiology lies within the fourth and final compartment of the hip, the iliopsoas compartment.

Patrick's Test - Variation Two. In the FABER position, place hand on medial aspect of knee have patient externally rotate against resistance .

Positive Test: Anterior or medial groin pain or weakness.

Indicates: May represent iliopsoas insufficiency or pathology.

Psoas Test. Performed with the hip flexed to 30° while the patient attempts to raise the knee against resistance (Figure 7.24).

Positive Test: Pain at the lesser trochanteric region or may elicit a snapping sound at the internal hip. Hip extension (stretching of the iliopsoas) exacerbates the symptoms.

Indicates: Psoas muscle pathology.

Thomas Test - BASIC EXAM. Performed supine. Stabilize pelvis with one hand supporting lumbar spine, patient flexes one knee to the chest, opposite leg is extended (Figure 7.25). Repeat on other side for comparison.

Positive Test: Extended leg rises off the table.

Indicates: Hip Flexor (usually psoas) contraction.

COMMON CONDITIONS (Table 7.4)

Differential Diagnosis

The differential diagnosis for hip pathology includes many different entities and not uncommonly,

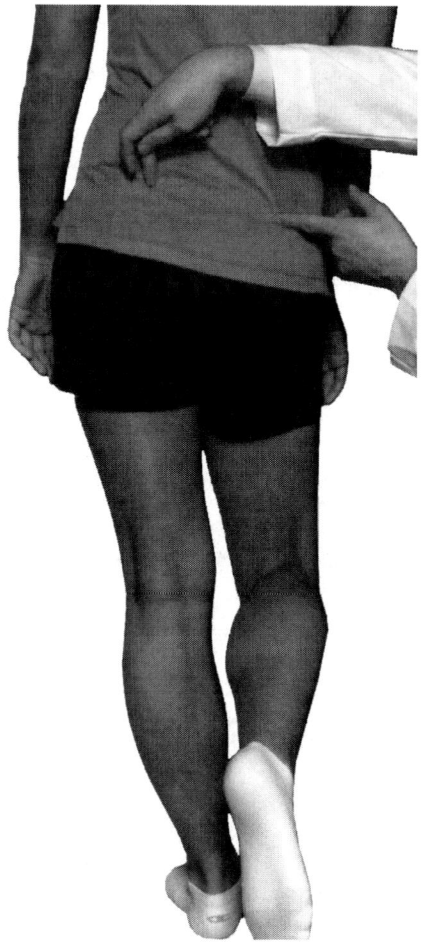

Figure 7.23. Positive Trendelenburg Test on the left.

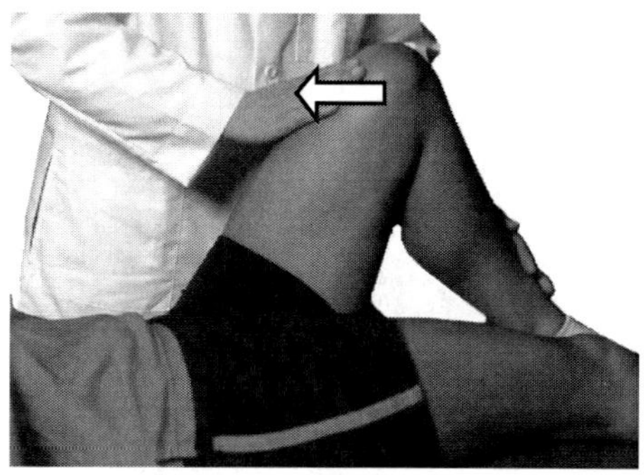

Figure 7.24. Psoas Test.

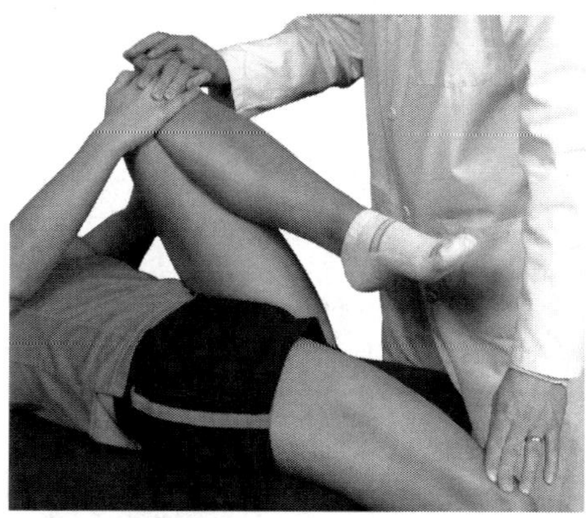

Figure 7.25. Thomas Test.

Table 7.4. Common Conditions.

Compartment	Conditions
<u>1: Central Compartment</u> 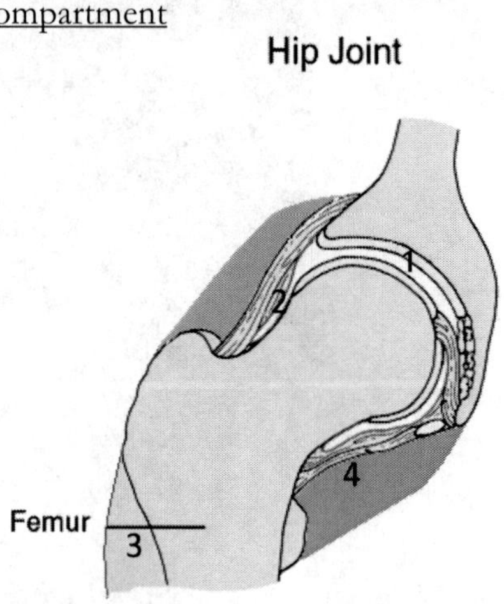	Labral tears Ligament Teres tears Osteochondral defects Chondromalacia/ Osteoarthritis Congenital Hip Dysplasia Loose Bodies
<u>2: Peripheral Compartment</u>	Loose Bodies Impingement syndrome Pincer Type CAM Type Synovitis
<u>3: Lateral Compartment</u>	Iliotibial (IT) Band Syndrome Bursitis Rotator cuff Tendonopathies Gluteus Medius Gluteus Minimus Piriformis
<u>4: Iliopsoas Bursae Compartment</u>	Psoas Tendonitis

multiple diagnoses are contributing to the patient's pain. Often, a peripheral, or causation etiology, is diagnosed and the underlying primary lesion remains undiscovered. Therefore, it is important to consider these referred pain patterns in the differential diagnosis to reduce inappropriate testing.[12]

CONDITIONS THAT SHOULD NOT BE MISSED DUE TO POSSIBLE MORBIDITY OR MORTALITY

Compartmental infection should be suspected in all cases where fever is concomitant with pain on range of motion or with weight bearing.

Hip fracture and dislocation are usually associated with high-velocity trauma such as seen in a motor vehicle accident or other rapid decelerating injury. Pain is markedly increased with weight bearing or log roll on evaluation. Congenital hip dysplasia is a disorder in children that is either present at birth or shortly thereafter. The acetabulum should cover the head of the femur and hold it in place by the socket deepening labral rim. In the event of congenital hip dysplasia, the development of the acetabulum in an infant allows the femoral head to ride upward out of the joint socket, especially when weight bearing begins.

Displaced fractures of the femoral neck are more common in individuals over 60 years of age. Osteoporosis is a major contributing factor and is therefore more common in women due to their predisposition to this condition. Avascular necrosis is a condition that results in the collapse of the matrix of the femoral head. This occurs due to traumatic disruption of the delicate arterial supply in this region. A simple fall or sudden distraction of the joint may be all that it takes to initiate this condition.

Slipped capital femoral epiphysis is found in older children and adolescents. The presenting complaint is often a limping child with knee pain. The epiphysis progressively displaces from microtrauma exposing a weakened ossification.

Trochanteric pain may be due to mass occupying lesions such as calcific tendinopathy, tuberculosis, giant cell carcinoma, and rheumatoid inflammation of the trochanteric bursa.[9-12] Hemorrhagic bursitis following an acute fall and infectious bursitis must also be considered.[12] Calcific bursitis is thought to occur due to dystrophic calcium deposition into the collagen matrix due to chronic imflammation.[13]

Adiposa Dolorosa is a pain syndrome in the subcutaneous fatty tissue at the lateral aspect of the hip.[6] Typically, these patients are morbidly obese and pain is elicited on palpation of the fatty tissues rather than with palpation of the trochanteric bursa.

Psuedoradiculopathies can result in upper lateral thigh pain and are referred from the nociceptive fibers of the lumbar roots, facet joints and paraspinous ligaments.[6] The iliohypogastric nerve and subcostal nerves are the most common nerve entrapments in the hip region. The most common site of entrapment of the iliohypogastric nerve is approximately 10cm posterior to the anterior superior iliac spine. At this level, the nerve crosses the iliac crest.[6] The subcostal nerves can be trapped more posterior over the brim of the iliac crest.[6] The lateral femoral cutaneous nerve can also refer pain to the lateral aspect of the thigh. The pain in this case is often more anterior than lateral.[6]

REFERENCES

1. Shbeeb MI, Matteson EL. Trochanteric bursitis (greater trochanter pain syndrome). *Mayo Clin Proc.* Jun 1996;71(6):565-569.
2. Spear IM LP. Noninfectious trochanteric bursitis and peritendinitis. *Surg Clin North Am.* 1952;32:1217-1224.
3. Collee G, Dijkmans BA, Vandenbroucke JP, Cats A. Greater trochanteric pain syndrome (trochanteric bursitis) in low back pain. *Scand J Rheumatol.* 1991;20(4):262-266.
4. Larsson LG, Baum J. The syndromes of bursitis. *Bull Rheum Dis.* 1986;36:1-8.
5. Tanaka H, Kido K, Wakisaka A, Mine T, Kawai S. Trochanteric bursitis in rheumatoid arthritis. *J Rheumatol.* Jun 2002;29(6):1340-1341.
6. Traycoff RB. "Pseudotrochanteric bursitis": the differential diagnosis of lateral hip pain. *J Rheumatol.* Dec 1991;18(12):1810-1812.
7. Kingzett-Taylor A, Tirman PF, Feller J, et al. Tendinosis and tears of gluteus medius and minimus muscles as a cause of hip pain: MR imaging findings. *AJR Am J Roentgenol.* Oct 1999;173(4):1123-1126.
8. Swezey RL. Pseudo-radiculopathy in subacute trochanteric bursitis of the subgluteus maximus bursa. *Arch Phys Med Rehabil.* Aug 1976;57(8):387-390.
9. Leonard MH. Trochanteric syndrome; calcareous and noncalcareous tendonitis and bursitis about the trochanter major. *J Am Med Assoc.* Sep 13 1958;168(2):175-177.
10. Willson JD, Dougherty CP, Ireland ML, Davis IM. Core stability and its relationship to lower extremity function and injury. *J Am Acad Orthop Surg.* Sep 2005;13(5):316-325.
11. Raman D, Haslock I. Trochanteric bursitis--a frequent cause of 'hip' pain in rheumatoid arthritis. *Ann Rheum Dis.* Dec 1982;41(6):602-603.
12. Wakeshima Y, Ellen MI. Atypical hip pain origin in a young athletic woman: a case report of giant cell carcinoma. *Arch Phys Med Rehabil.* Oct 2001;82(10):1472-1475.
13. Schein AJ, Lehmann O. Acute trochanteric bursitis with calcification. *Surgery.* 1941;9:771-779.
14. Dougherty C, Dougherty J. Evaluating hip pathology in trochanteric pain syndrome. *J Musculoskeletal Med.* 2008;25.

8

The Knee Exam

Michael Henehan, D.O., FAOASM

Craig Phelps, D.O., FAOASM

Lee Rice, D.O., FAOASM

ANATOMY

Bones

The knee primarily functions as a hinge joint with the articulation between the femur and the tibia serving as the main load bearing and pivot surfaces. At the distal end of the femur the bone widens to form two rounded structures called the medial and lateral femoral condyles. These provide load bearing over the full range of motion (approximately 150 degrees) of the knee. The condyles, as a function of their rounded shape, also allow for limited rotational movement as well. The proximal tibia provides a flat surface upon which the femoral condyles rest. In the healthy knee joint the distal femur and proximal tibial articular surfaces are covered with hyaline cartilage. This provides an exceptionally smooth surface that allows for easy movement of the knee. The two other bones in the knee joint, the patella and the fibula, also play significant biomechanical roles.

The patella is a large sesamoid bone that functions as the insertion of the quadriceps tendon and the origin of the infrapatellar ligament. It provides anterior stabilization and allows smooth transmission of force from the quadriceps muscle to its attachment at the distal end of the tibia on the anterior tibial tuberosity. The patellofemoral joint is the articulation between the posterior patella and the anterior portions of the femoral condyles. This joint allows for the knee to move as a hinge while the quadriceps muscles provide the power to extend the knee.

The fibula acts as a strut to allow rotation of the lower leg without sacrificing stability. The proximal end or fibular head articulates medially with the lateral portion of the tibial plateau. This is a synovial, condyloid joint, supported by a fibrous capsule with anterior and posterior ligaments encircling the joint.

Muscles

There are two main muscle groups that act on the knee. These are collectively called the knee extensors and the knee flexors.

The extensors include the quadriceps and tensor fascia latae muscles. The quadriceps consists of the vastus medialis, vastus intermedius, vastus lateralis and rectus femoris. The quadriceps muscles attach on the superior pole of the patella. The force of these muscles then act through the patella on the infrapatellar ligament and its attachment to the anterior tibial tuberosity.

The primary knee flexors consist of the hamstring muscles - semitendinosis, gracilis and long head of the biceps femoris. All of these muscles cross the hip and act as extensors of the hip as well. The short head of the biceps does not cross the hip, but still acts as a knee flexor. The gastrocnemius and plantaris are also knee flexors. The gracilis works to adduct the hip and flex the knee. The sartorius is also a weak knee flexor. The semitendinosis, gracilis and sartorius insert as a common tendon on the medial aspect of the proximal tibia becoming what is known as the pes anserinus.

Table 8.1. Muscles of the Knee

Knee Flexors	Origin	Insertion	Innervation
Biceps femoris, long head	Ischial tuberosity	Lateral condyle of tibia and fibular head	Tibial nerve
Biceps femoris, short head	Lateral linea aspera of femur	Lateral condyle of tibia	Common peroneal nerve
Gracilis (weak flexor)	Lower symphysis Pubic arch	Upper medial tibia	Obturator
Popliteus	Lateral condyle of femur	Posterior tibia above soleal line	Tibial nerve
Semimembranosis	Lower medial ischial tuberosity	Medial body of tibia	Tibial nerve
Semitendinosis	Upper outer ischial tuberosity	Posterior medial aspect of tibial condyle	Tibial nerve
Sartorius	Anterior superior iliac spine	Upper medial tibia	Femoral nerve
Gastrocnemius	Upper posterior medial femoral condyle	Posterior calcaneus	Tibial nerve
Plantaris	Lower lateral femoral supracondylar line	Posterior calcaneus	Tibial nerve
Knee Extensors	**Origin**	**Insertion**	**Innervation**
Rectus femoris	Anterior inferior iliac spine and rim of acetabulum	Base of patella	Femoral nerve
Vastus lateralis	Intertrochanteric line of femur	Lateral patella	Femoral nerve
Vastus medius	Intertrochanteric line of femur	Medial patella	Femoral nerve
Vastus intermedius	Upper anterior shaft of femur	Base of patella	Femoral nerve
Tensor fascia lata	Anterior iliac crest	Superior lateral tibia through the Iliotibial band	Superior gluteal nerve

Ligaments

The knee contains several important ligamentous structures. The anterior cruciate ligament (ACL) originates in the posterior aspect of the lateral femoral condyle and attaches to the front of the tibial intercondylar eminence. The ACL functions to check extension, lateral rotation and anterior slipping of the tibia on the femur. The posterior cruciate ligament (PCL) originates on the anterior and lateral side of the medial femoral condyle and attaches to the posterior intercondylar fossa of the tibia. The PCL functions to check extension, lateral rotation and posterior slipping of the tibia on the femur. The medial collateral ligament (MCL) originates on the medial aspect of the medial femoral epicondyle and inserts on the medial aspect of the proximal tibia. It serves to limit valgus movement of the knee. The lateral collateral ligament (LCL) originates on the lateral aspect of the lateral femoral condyle and inserts on the lateral aspect of the proximal tibia. It serves to limit varus movement of the knee.

Meniscus

The medial and lateral menisci are "C" shaped cartilaginous structures that are attached to the tibial plateau by the menisco-tibial ligaments. They primarily help stabilize the femoral-tibial articulation, but may also help with weight transfer, knee proprioception and nutritional functions for the articular cartilage.

Nerves

The sciatic nerve divides into the posterior tibial nerve, which moves through the posterior fossa of the knee and the common peroneal nerve which courses laterally and branches into the superficial peroneal and sural nerves. The superficial peroneal nerve is subject to trauma as it courses anteriorly to the fibular head.

Arteries

The femoral artery divides into the popliteal artery, which courses through the popliteal fossa adjacent to the popliteal nerve and vein, and the genicular artery.

HISTORY AND PHYSICAL EXAMINATION

The examination always begins with a thorough history. This leads to a specific physical examination with provocative tests/maneuvers for evaluation of the suspected condition. It is recommended to examine the uninjured knee first. This allows the examiner to feel the "normal" ligaments first so there can be a comparison with the injured side. It also helps to put the patient at ease and helps them relax when examining the injured side.

Key Components of the Patient History

There are several clinical clues in evaluation of the knee that provide consistently helpful information and should be part of any knee evaluation. A history of a "pop" followed by immediate swelling (within 4 hours) is strongly suggestive of an anterior cruciate ligament tear. Clicking, locking and recurrent swelling should make the examiner think of a possible meniscus tear. Bilateral knee pain, particularly in an adolescent female, is suggestive of an overuse or biomechanical problem such as a subluxing patella or patellofemoral pain syndrome.

Observation

It is helpful to note if the patient has an abnormal gait, limp, bruising, abrasions or obvious deformity to the knee. Large effusions can be noted on inspection, particularly in thin individuals. An effusion extending into the popliteal fossa is known as a Baker's cyst. It is also important to look at the position of the patella. The patella usually is centered directly over the joint. When it is higher than usual it is called patella alta. Lower than normal is patella baja. There can also be lateral displacement or a lateral tilt to the patella, which may suggest patellar subluxation. The position of the tibia relative to the femur is important to note. Genu valgum (knock-knees), genu varum (bowlegs) and genu recurvatum (hyperextension) should be noted. If appropriate, x-rays can be used to take measurements of the knee articulation.

Palpation

Palpation of the knee should be completed in a systematic manner with close attention to anatomical details. There is no "one way" to position a patient for a knee exam. One option is to have the patient prone with the knee flexed to 90 degrees. It is helpful to approach the exam by dividing the knee into four regions: anterior, medial, lateral and posterior.

Anterior: Start by palpating for a joint effusion. If there is a large effusion it is usually easy to feel the fluid when comparing one knee to the other. More subtle effusions can be detected by compressing the suprapatellar pouch of the joint. This pushes the fluid to down, stretching out the joint capsule much like squeezing a water balloon in one area causes it to bulge out elsewhere. This maneuver also helps to distinguish swelling of the pre-patella bursa, which remains fixed in the pre-patellar area with compression. It is also important to note if the joint is warm to touch as this can indicate inflammation or possibly infection.

Palpate the anterior tibial tuberosity, infrapatellar tendon, the body of the patella and the suprapatellar tendon. Note tenderness or swelling.

Posterior: Palpate the popliteal fossa noting effusion extending into the fossa (Baker's cyst) or bone irregularity. Occasionally a bone tumor called an osteochondroma can be found in this area. Tenderness along the posterior joint lines may indicate meniscal injury. The popliteus tendon can be palpated at the lateral femoral origin and tibial attachment. The popliteal artery can be palpated as well.

Medial: Palpate the joint line. Tenderness in this area is suggestive of a meniscus tear. Tenderness or focal swelling above or below the joint line is suggestive of an MCL sprain. Just slightly posterior and inferior to the MCL attachment is the pes anserinus and its associated bursa. Tenderness here can indicate pes anserine bursitis.

Lateral: Palpate the lateral joint line and lateral collateral ligament as was done on the medial side. Palpate the fibular head and the attachment of the biceps femoris. The superficial peroneal nerve runs posterior to the fibular head. Normally the nerve is not palpable. Palpate the iliotibial band and its attachment on the lateral tibia at Gerdy's tubercle. Grasp the fibular head with the thumb and index finger to check motion and to diagnose anterior or posterior fibular head somatic dysfunction.

Neurovascular Examination

In an acute knee injury, the neurovascular exam should be performed quickly to assess nerve damage and vascular compromise before any provocative tests are done. Evidence of nerve or vascular damage constitutes a medical emergency and urgent orthopedic consultation is indicated.

Vascular: Palpate the popliteal artery in the popliteal fossa. The pulse should be equal bilaterally. Assess bilateral distal pulses (dorsal pedis and posterior tibial) as well. **NOTE: In severe knee trauma, such as a dislocation, popliteal artery rupture must be ruled out.**

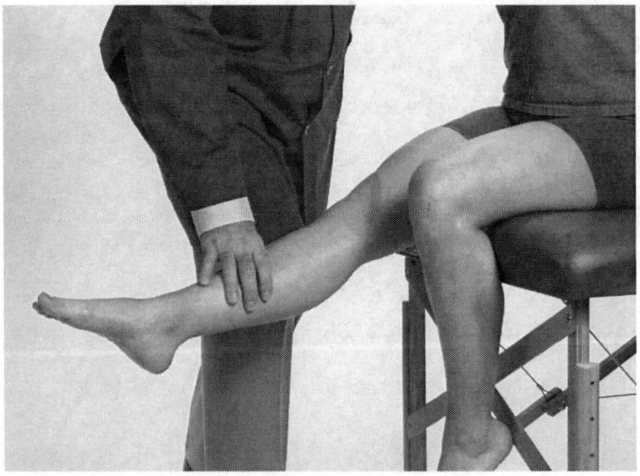

Figure 8.1. Testing quadriceps strength.

Neuro: The patellar tendon reflex can be checked with the patient in the seated position. Sensation should be checked around the knee joint.

Muscle Strength Testing

Whenever possible, test muscle strength bilaterally and simultaneously to detect subtle strength differences.

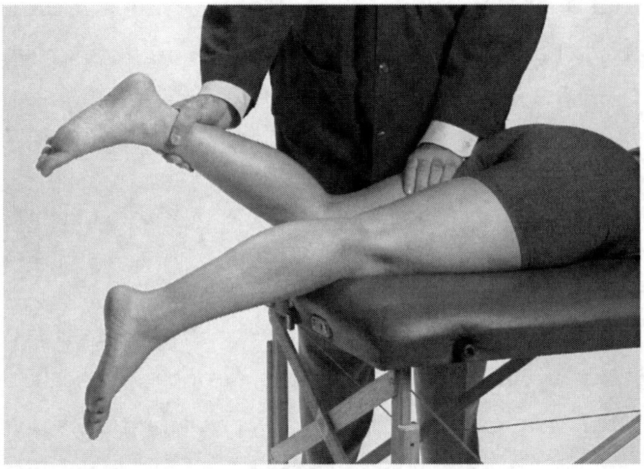

Figure 8.2. Testing hamstring strength in prone position.

Quadriceps: It is easiest to test this muscle group with the patient in the sitting position. The examiner places his/her hand against the patient's anterior tibial surface while the patient's knee is flexed to 90 degrees. The patient then extends the leg(s) against the resisting force applied by the examiner (Figure 8.1).

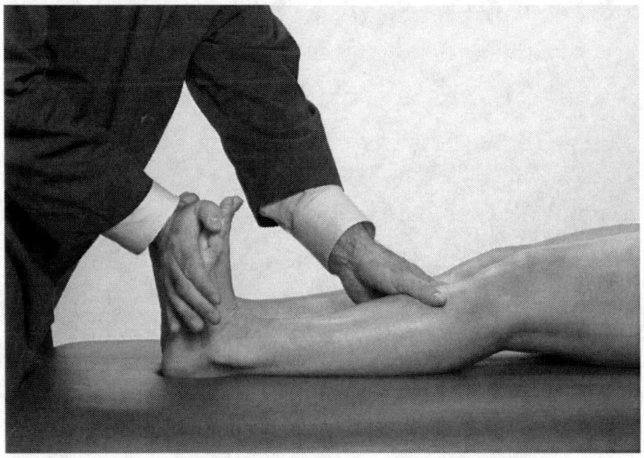

Figure 8.3. Testing gastrocnemius strength.

Hamstring: With the patient in the sitting position and the knees flexed to 90 degrees, the examiner places his or her hand on the posterior aspect of the lower leg and asks the patient to flex the knee with a resisting force applied by the examiner. This test can also be done with the patient in a prone position (Figure 8.2).

Gastrocnemius: Start with the patient in the supine position, with the knee resting in the extended position and the foot 0 degrees plantar flexed. The examiner places his hand on the plantar surface of the foot and has the patient plantar flex the foot against the examiners resistance (Figure 8.3).

Range of Motion

The knee functions primarily as a hinge joint with a normal range of motion between 145 – 150 degrees of flexion and 0 – 5 degrees of extension. Varus and valgus motion is normally limited to a few degrees and should be bilaterally symmetrical.

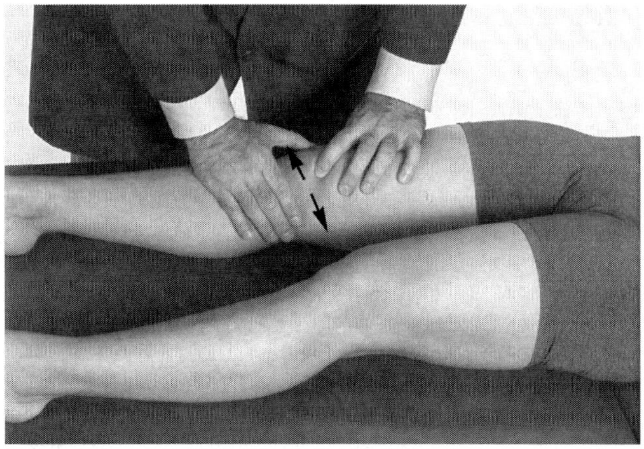

Figure 8.4. Patellar Laxity and Apprehension Tests.

It is important to assess the quality of the range of motion. Feel for ease of motion and crepitus in the knee through the full range of motion. Crepitus or catching of the patella may indicate chondromalacia patella or osteoarthritis.

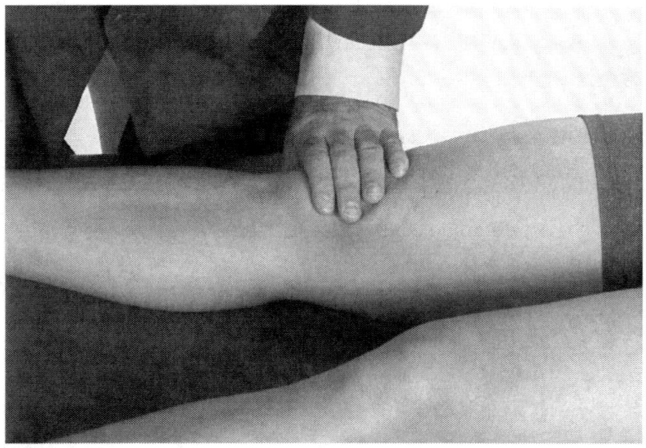

Figure 8.5. Patellar Compression (Grind) Test.

Patellar mobility: When passively testing patellar motion observe the movement of the patella as it articulates with the femur. The patella should start laterally in full extension, move medially into the sulcus during mid-range of flexion and then move laterally as the knee is fully flexed.

PROVOCATIVE TESTS AND MANEUVERS

Patellar Mechanism

Patellar Laxity Test. The examiner positions one hand above and one hand below the joint. The thumbs are placed against the medical aspect of the patella. The examiner then pushes the patella laterally, assessing the range of motion (Figure 8.4). Laxity can be described on a 1-4 scale using the body of the patella as its own measurement tool. Excursion of 0-25% the width of the patella is considered +1, 25-50% equals +2, 50-75% equals +3 and > 75% equals +4.

Patellar Apprehension Test. This is basically a continuation of the patellar laxity test. When testing patellar laxity to the point of restriction, ask the patient if the maneuver provokes any discomfort or sensation of instability. A positive sense of apprehension or instability indicates possible previous patellar dislocation or severe instability.

Patellar (Grind) Compression Test. With the patient in the supine position, and the knee extended, the examiner provides a compressive load to the patella with one hand (Figure 8.5) while moving the patella medial and lateral.

Positive Test: Pain with compression.

Indicates: Possible inflammation, chondromalacia, or injury to the patellofemoral articular surfaces.

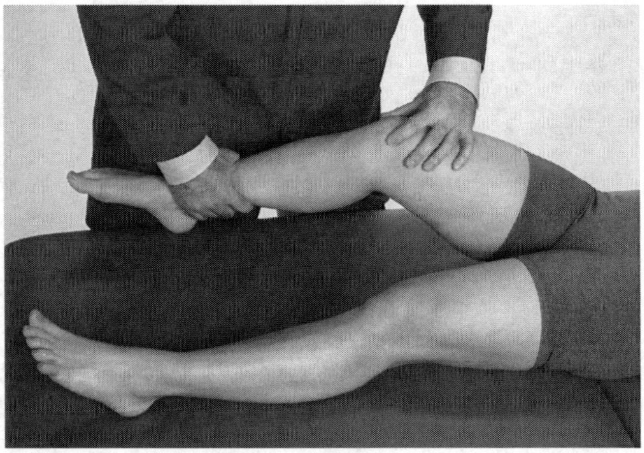

Figure 8.6. Patellar Glide Test.

Patellar Glide Test. With the patient in a sitting or supine position have him or her slowly extend and flex the knee and note the quality of the articular motion as previously described in the range of motion section. Having the examiner place his hand lightly over the patella can increase the sensitivity of the test (Figure 8.6).

Positive Test: Palpable or audible crepitus, pain or catching of the patella

Indicates: Possible damage to the articular surface.

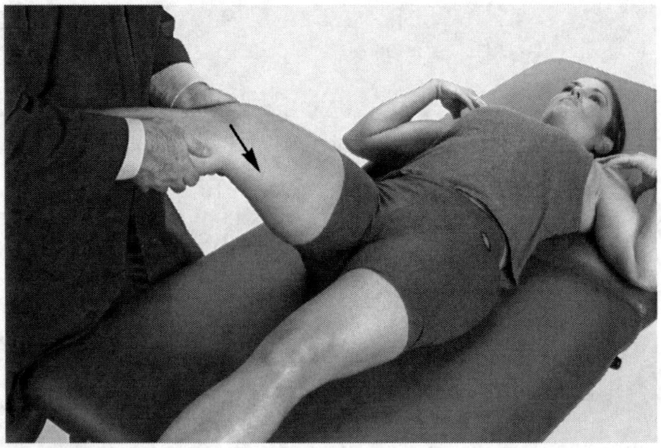

Figure 8.7. Valgus Stress Test at 30 degrees of knee flexion.

Collateral Ligaments

Valgus Stress Test (Knee at 30 Degrees of Flexion). With the patient in the supine position, the examiner supports the patient's lower leg on the examiner's hip holding it in place with the forearm. The examiner's hands are then placed on the medial and lateral aspects of the patient's knee. The examiner then moves the lower leg so that the ankle shifts laterally while holding the distal femur in place (Figure 8.7). This creates a valgus load on the medial collateral ligament of the knee. The test is done in 30 degrees flexion and neutral. The examiner assess for laxity, quality of end point and pain.

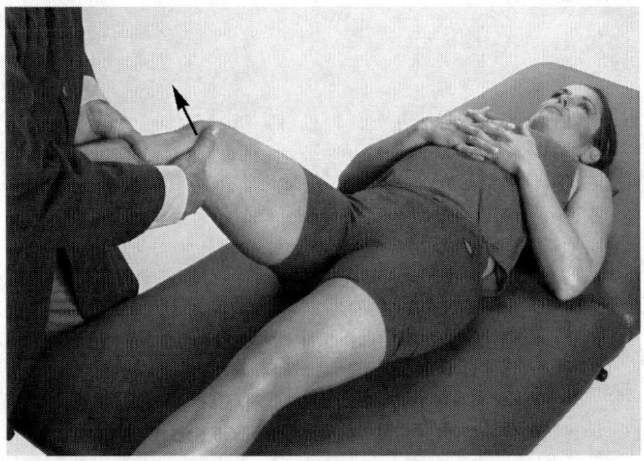

Figure 8.8. Varus Stress Test at 30 degrees of knee flexion.

Positive Test: Increased laxity, soft or absent endpoint or pain.

Indicates: Medial collateral ligament disruption.

Valgus Stress Test (Knee at 0 Degrees of Flexion). The positioning of patient and examiner is the same except for the degree of knee flexion.

Positive Test: Laxity.

Indicates: More severe injury possibly including the posterior joint capsule, anterior cruciate ligament and medial collateral ligament.

Varus Stress Test. The examiner and patient's positioning is the same as for the ***Valgus Stress Test.*** The examiner then moves the lower leg so that the ankle shifts medially while holding the distal femur in place (Figure 8.8). This creates a varus load on the lateral collateral ligament of the knee. The test is done in 30 degrees flexion and neutral. Findings indicate the similar pathology as with valgus loading, but specific to the lateral collateral ligament and lateral joint capsule.

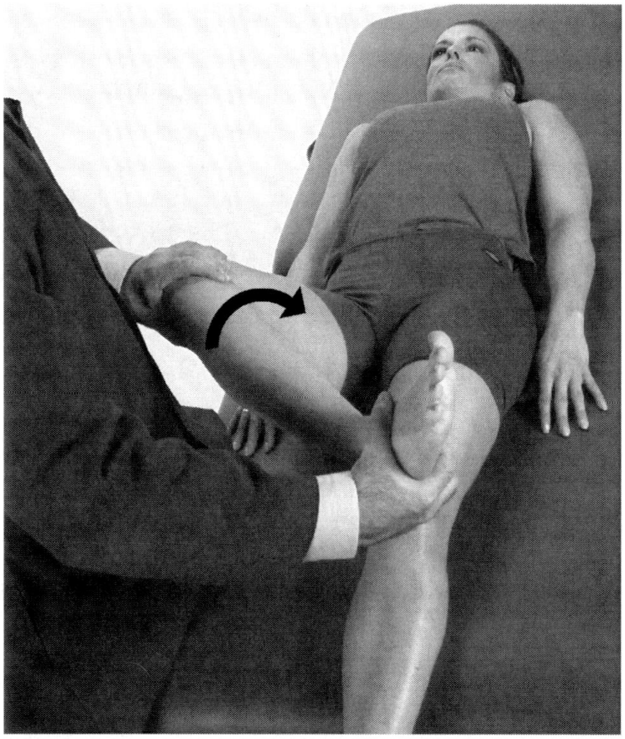

Figure 8.9. McMurray's Test stressing the medial meniscus.

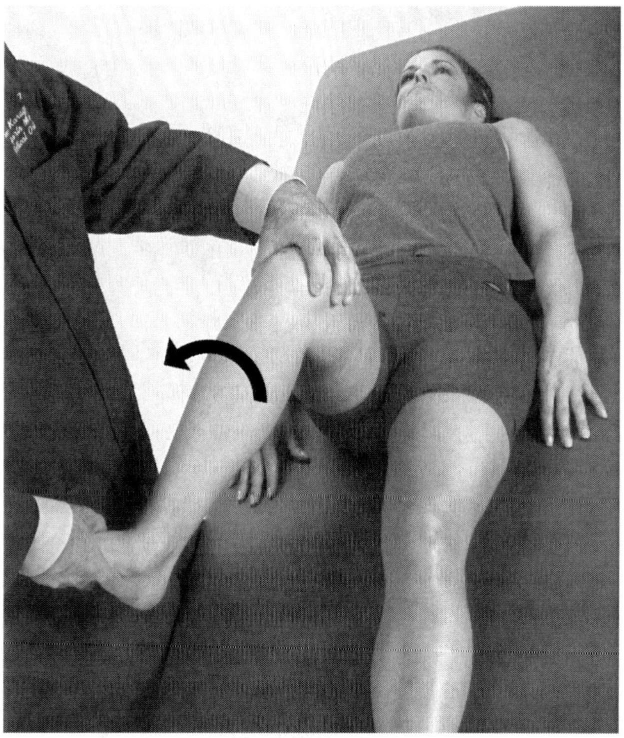

Figure 8.10. McMurray's Test stressing the lateral meniscus.

Meniscus

McMurray's Test. The purpose of the test is to pinch the torn meniscus between the tibial plateau and femoral condyles. The examiner lifts the leg of the supine patient, one hand controlling the ankle while the other controls the distal femur. The knee is then flexed. To stress the medial meniscus, the tibia is internally rotated as the knee is extended while adding a varus load. The examiner is stressing the tibia medially so as to compress the medial joint compartment, while the rotation forces the condyles on and against the medial meniscus (Figure 8.9).

Positive Test: Pain or a painful click while the knee is brought into extension.

Indicates: Possible meniscus tear.

To test the lateral meniscus, the positioning of the hands remains the same but the application of force is reversed. That is, the knee is flexed and an external rotation of the tibia with a valgus load added while the knee is brought back into extension (Figure 8.10). A positive test is the same as the medial and also indicates a possible meniscal tear.

Bounce Test. The clinician takes the relaxed supine leg with one hand on the proximal tibia and the other on the ankle. The clinician first raises the knee about 6 inches, flexes the knee about 10 degrees and then lets the knee fall back into extension. The key is to perform this in a relaxed fashion with only a minimum of force.

Positive Test: Pain when the knee fully extends (on the bounce).

Indicates: Possible meniscus pathology.

Apley's Grind Test. The patient is prone with the knee flexed to 90 degrees. The clinician pushes down on the foot to provide a compression force on the meniscus while rotating the foot internally and externally (Figure 8.11). The maneuver is then repeated with a distraction force pulling up on the foot.

Positive Test: Pain with rotation and/or compression.

Indicates: Pain during the compression plus rotation part of the test could be meniscus injury, collateral ligament injury or both. Pain with the distraction plus rotation part of the test indicates collateral ligament damage.

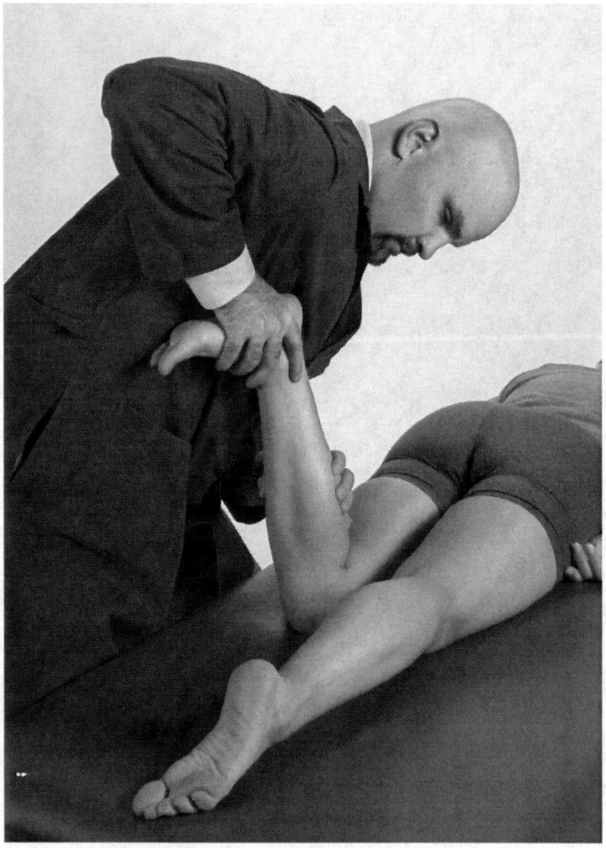

Figure 8.11. Apley's Grind Test.

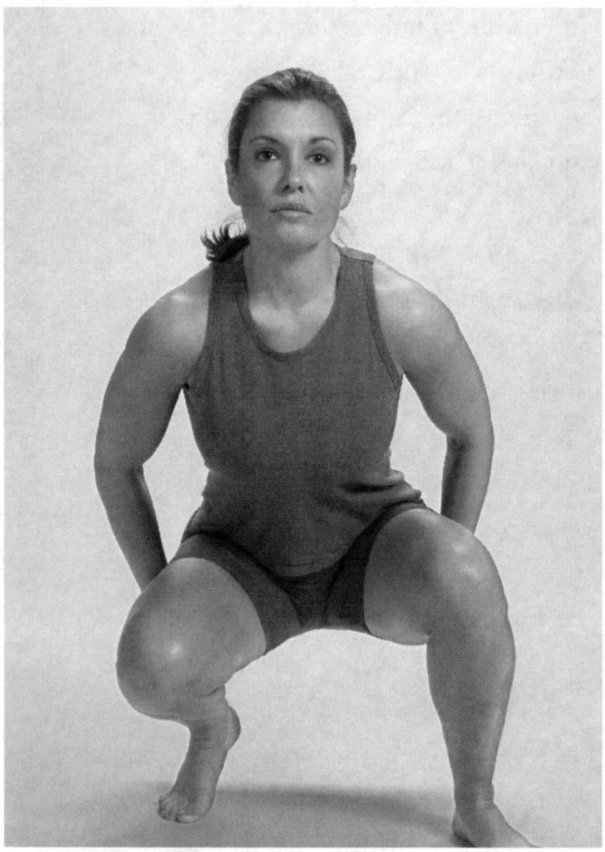

Figure 8.12. Duck Walk Test.

Squat or Duck Walk Test. The patient squats and attempts to walk in a squatting position (Figure 8.12). (Caution: this test produces a significant load on the meniscus and patellofemoral joint and may cause further damage to these structures. The test should not be performed if there is a high level of suspicion for a meniscus tear as further damage to the meniscus can occur. It acts as a screening test for knee pathology.)

Positive Test: Knee pain.

Indicates: Meniscus tear or patellofemoral joint inflammation.

Anterior Stability

Lachman's Test. While the patient is supine, the clinician places the proximal stabilizing hand on the distal thigh just above the patella. The distal mobilizing hand grasps the proximal tibia. Flexing the knee to 30 degrees, the examiner uses his distal hand to pull the tibia anteriorly while the proximal hand stabilizes the thigh (Figure 8.13).

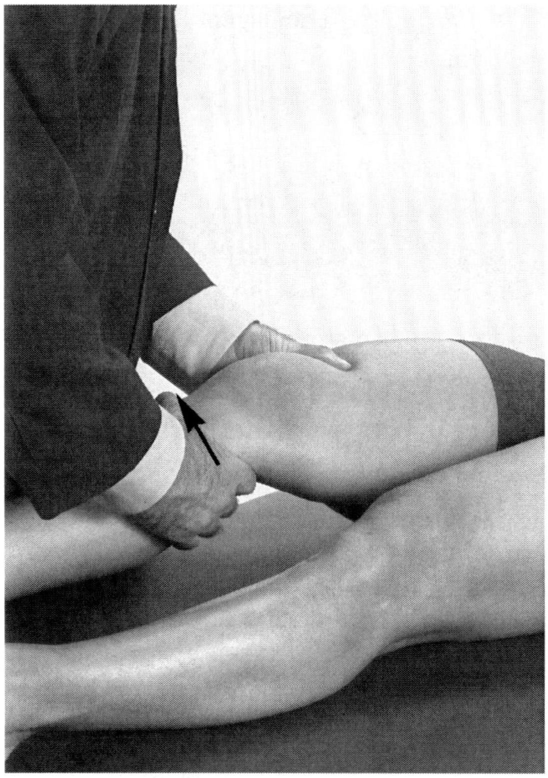

Figure 8.13. Lachman's Test.

Positive Test: Increased laxity, soft or absent end point.

Indicates: Anterior cruciate ligament insufficiency.

Anterior Drawer Test. The patient is positioned in the supine position with the knee flexed to 90 degrees. The clinician sits on the patient's foot to stabilize the leg while the examiner grasps the proximal tibia with both hands and pulls the tibia anteriorly (Figure 8.14).

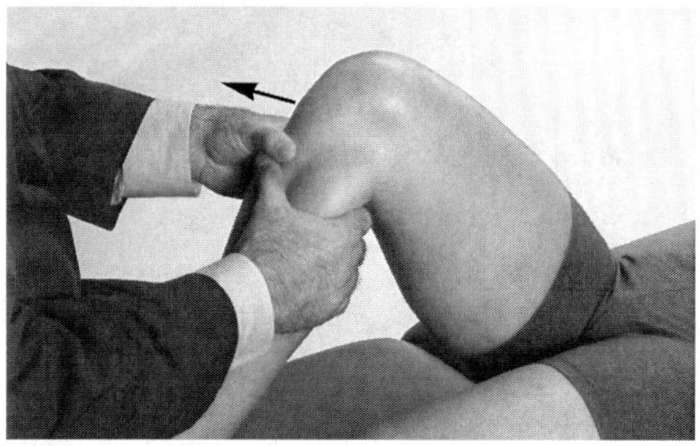

Figure 8.14. Anterior Drawer Test.

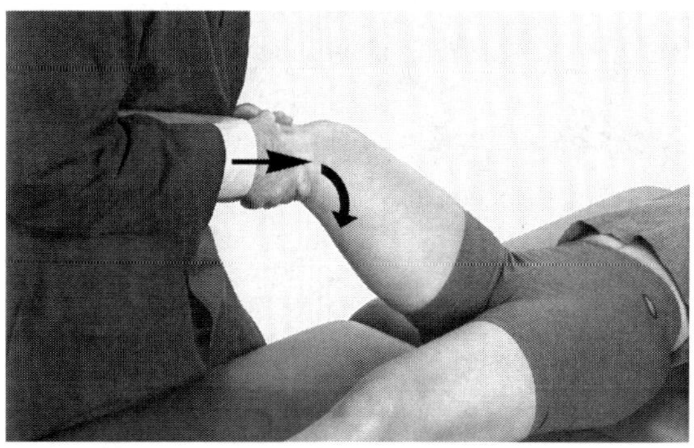

Figure 8.15. Pivot Shift Test.

Positive Test: Excessive translation when compared to the other knee.

Indicates: Anterior cruciate ligament insufficiency.

Pivot Shift Test. The patient is supine while the clinician holds the knee with both hands. The knee is held in 20 degrees of flexion and neutral rotation. The patient is asked to relax the leg, which allows the femur to sag back when the anterior cruciate ligament is disrupted. The knee is then moved into extension while applying a valgus force. The knee is flexed to 40 degrees, causing the forward subluxation of the tibia during the sudden change in direction (Figure 8.15). The test can be difficult to do since it is hard for the patient to relax during the exam.

Positive Test: Tibial subluxation at 20 to 40 degrees of flexion, shifting or "clunking" of the tibia against the femur.

Indicates: Anterior cruciate ligament deficiency.

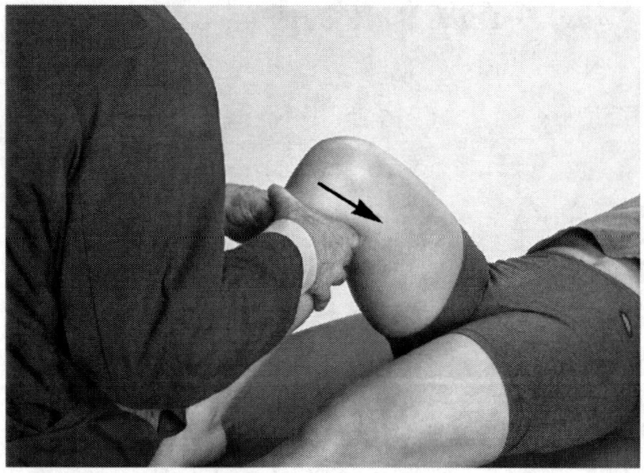

Figure 8.16. Posterior Drawer Test.

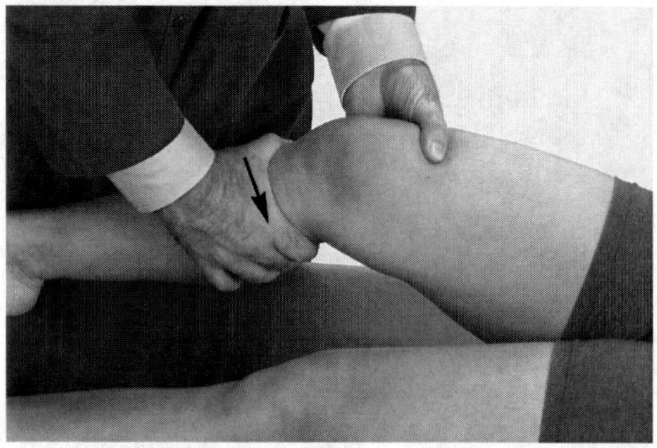

Figure 8.17. Reverse Lachman's Test.

Posterior Stability

Posterior Drawer Test. The knee is positioned the same as for the anterior drawer test. The clinician grasps the knee and translates the tibia in a posterior direction (Figure 8.16).

Positive Test: Excessive translation, particularly when compared to the opposite side.

Indicates: Posterior cruciate ligament deficiency, posterior capsular injury or disruption.

Sag Test. Both knees are positioned as for the anterior drawer test and the prominence of the anterior tibial plateau is assessed for bilateral symmetry.

Positive Test: The tibial plateau of the affected side sags posterior when compared to the uninjured side.

Indicates: Posterior cruciate ligament deficiency.

EDITOR'S NOTE: All of the Provocative Tests up to this point are part of the Basic Knee Exam that should be performed on every patient with knee complaints. The remainder of the tests are specific for patients with a history of a mechanism of injury suggesting possible PCL/posterior capsule injury or complaints of posterolateral knee pain.

Reverse Lachman's Test. The position of the hands and knee are the same as for Lachman's Test. The proximal hand stabilizes the femur while the distal hand pushes the tibia posterior (Figure 8.17).

Positive Test: Increased laxity, soft or absent end point when compared to the opposite joint.

Indicates: Posterior cruciate ligament deficiency or posterior capsule deficiency.

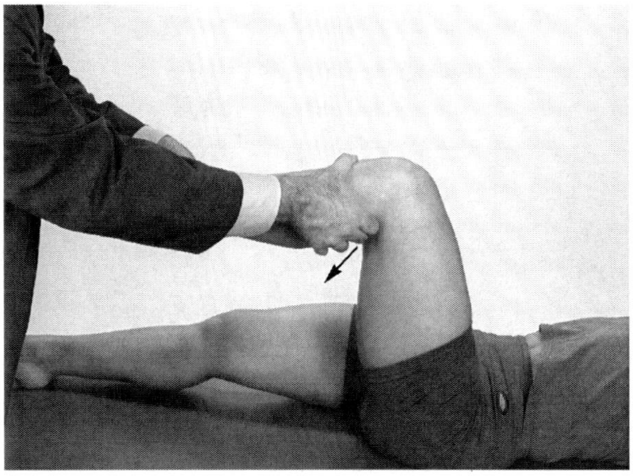

Figure 8.18. Dynamic Posterior Shift Test.

Quadriceps Active Test. This test is most effective when the sag test is positive. The patient's knee is flexed to 60 degrees and the examiner secures the foot on the table. The patient attempts to extend the knee with an isometric contraction.

Positive Test: Anterior tibial translation, which recreates the 1-cm step off between the medial femoral condyle and the medial tibial plateau.

Indicates: Posterior cruciate ligament deficiency.

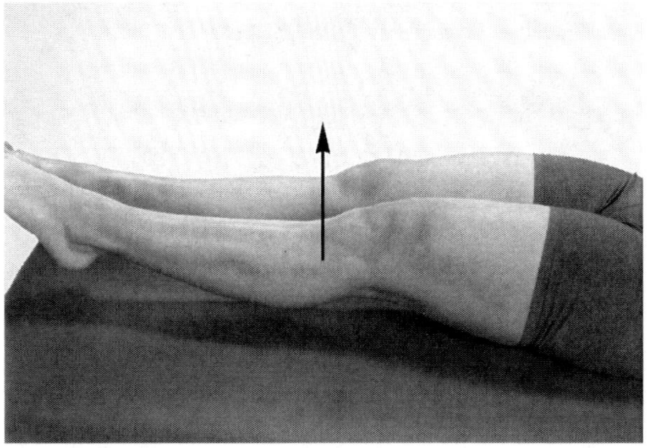

Figure 8.19. External Rotation Recurvatum Test.

Dynamic Posterior Shift Test. With the patient in the supine position, the knee and hip are flexed at 90 degrees. The patient slowly extends the knee to full extension. With posterior cruciate ligament deficiency, the tibia is subluxed posterior throughout its range of motion and then it is reduced at full extension (Figure 8.18).

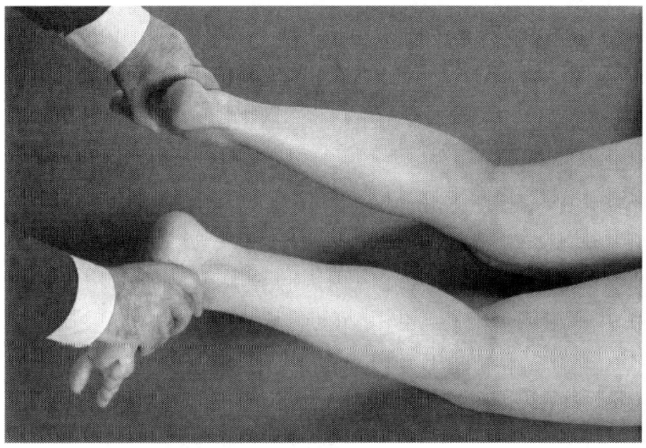

Figure 8.20. External Rotation Dial Test at 30 degrees of knee flexion.

Positive Test: Clunk near full extension.

Indicates: Posterior cruciate ligament deficiency.

External Rotation Recurvatum Test. The clinician lifts both supine legs by the great toes (Figure 8.19).

Positive Test: The knee drops into varus alignment and hyperextension compared to the uninjured side. Recurvatum bilaterally suggests generalized ligamentous laxity.

Indicates: Posterolateral instability, posterior cruciate ligament deficiency.

Posterior Capsule

External Rotation Dial Test. While the patient is prone, the feet are passively externally rotated, measuring rotation with the thigh –foot angle and comparing to the other side. Perform with the knee flexed in 30 (Figure 8.20) and 90 degrees of flexion (Figure 8.21).

Positive Test: 10-degree difference between the knees in 30 degrees of flexion.

Indicates: Possible posterior capsular disruption.

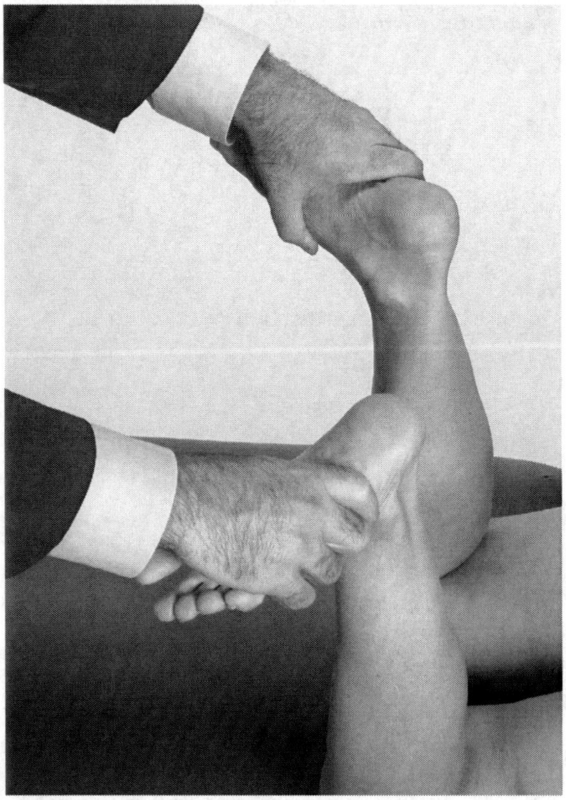

Figure 8.21. External Rotation Dial Test at 90 degrees of knee flexion.

Reverse Pivot Shift Test. With the patient supine, the examiner applies a valgus force to the knee flexed in 90 degrees. The knee is then slowly extended with the valgus force still applied (Figure 8.22).

Positive Test: Visible shift or clunk near 30 degrees of flexion.

Indicates: Poster lateral capsular injury or posterior cruciate ligament deficiency.

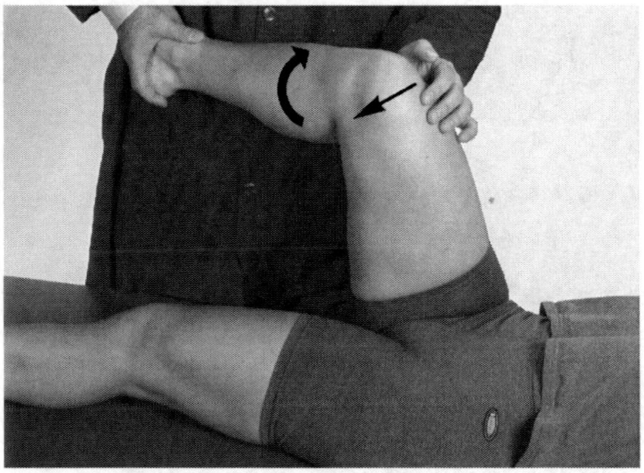

Figure 8.22. Reverse Pivot Shift Test.

Popliteus Muscle

Garrick's Test. While the patient lies supine the clinician flexes the hip and knee 90 degrees, internally rotating the lower leg. The patient holds the leg in this position while the examiner applies an external rotation resistance (Figure 8.23).

Positive Test: Pain with muscle contraction.

Indicates: Popliteus muscle injury/tendonitis.

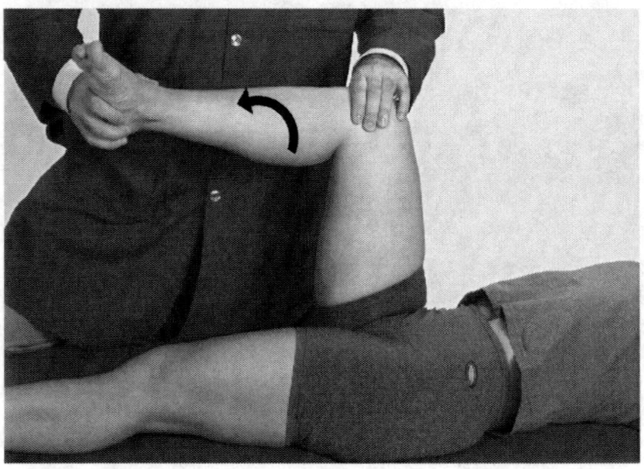

Figure 8.23. Garrick's Test for Popliteus Pathology.

COMMON CONDITIONS

- Ligament injury
  - Anterior cruciate
  - Posterior cruciate
  - Medial collateral
  - Lateral collateral
- Meniscal injury
  - Medial meniscus
  - Lateral meniscus
- Fractures:
  - Tibial plateau
  - Osteochondral
  - Patella
  - Femoral condyle
  - Fibular neck
- Overuse injuries
  - Patellofemoral syndrome
  - Iliotibial band friction syndrome
- Osteoarthritis
- Fibular head somatic dysfunction

CONDITIONS THAT SHOULD NOT BE MISSED DUE TO POSSIBLE MORBIDITY OR MORTALITY

- Fractures
- Infections
- Tumors
- Referred pain from the hip
- Popliteal artery rupture

REFERENCES

1. Hoppenfeld S. *Examination of the Spine and Extremities.* East Norwalk, CT: Appleton and Lange; 1976.
2. Karageanes SJ. *Principles of Manual Sports Medicine.* Philadelphia, PA: Lippincott Williams & Wilkins; 2005.

9
The Foot and Ankle Exam

R. Robert Franks, D.O., FAOASM

Kathryn C. Lambert, D.O.

ANATOMY

Bony Articulations

The ankle joint is formed from the articulation of the tibia, fibula and talus. The distal tibia widens to form the medial malleolus and the distal fibula widens to form the lateral malleolus. The lateral ankle has three ligaments arranged around the lateral malleolus that provide stability with inversion. They are from anterior to posterior, the anterior talofibular ligament, connecting the anterior aspect of the distal fibula and talar neck, the calcaneofibular ligament connecting the lateral malleolus and calcaneus, and the posterior talofibular ligament, connecting the posterior aspect of the distal fibula to the lateral talus. The medial ankle is supported by the deltoid ligament. The deltoid ligament is comprised of the following four ligaments arranged from anterior to posterior around the medial malleolus: the anterior tibiotalar ligament, the tibionavicular ligament, the tibiocalcaneal ligament, and the posterior tibiotalar ligament. The deltoid ligament connects the medial malleolus to the navicular, talus, and calcaneus. This ligament provides for stability with eversion and maintenance of the medial longitudinal foot arch.

The articulation of the tibia and fibula forms the tibiofibular joint. This joint is palpated directly above the talus and just medial to the lateral malleolus. The anterior and posterior inferior tibiofibular ligaments, referred to as the syndesmosis, provide stability at this joint. The syndesmosis is a tough fibrous connection that continues proximally to become the interosseus membrane. The interosseous membrane provides stability between the tibia and the fibula. The trochlea of the talus sits in the space referred to as the mortise, formed by the medial and lateral malleoli, which creates a hinge joint at the ankle itself. In plantar flexion, the talus moves anteriorly and in dorsiflexion it moves posteriorly.

The hindfoot is comprised of the calcaneus and talus and contains the subtalar joint formed by the articulation of these bones. Continuing distally, the hindfoot meets the midfoot, which contains the navicular, cuboid, and three cuneiform bones. Articulations here include the calcaneocuboid and the talocalcaneonavicular joint. These joints allow for inversion and eversion of the foot. As one continues through the midfoot, the transverse talar joint is formed by the articulation of the calcaneus and cuboid bone and talus and navicular bone.

Continuing distally, the forefoot contains the five metatarsal bones and all of the phalanges. The tarsometatarsal joint is formed between the medial, middle and lateral cuneiform bones, the cuboid bone and the metatarsals at the junction between the midfoot and forefoot. A fibrous capsule is formed at these joints by the dorsal, plantar, and interosseous ligaments. The first metatarsal is a critical bone as it bears the most weight and is necessary for propulsion during ambulation. The first metatarsal may have 2 sesamoid bones associated with it, which when present may be palpable. The metatarsals articulate with one another at their respective intermetatarsal joints. A fibrous capsule is formed at these joints again by the dorsal, plantar, and interosseous ligaments. The five metatarsals articulate with the five proximal phalanges forming the metatarsophalangeal joints. Fibrous capsules are formed at these joints by the collateral and plantar ligaments.

Finally, in toes two through five, the articulations between the proximal and middle phalanges are the proximal interphalangeal joints and the middle and distal phalanges are the distal interphalangeal joints. Having only 2 phalanges, the first toe has an interphalangeal joint and a metatarsophalangeal joint. All of these joints provide for flexion and extension of the toes. Again, there are fibrous capsules at these joints formed by the collateral and plantar ligaments. The skeletal articulations of the foot provide for not only the overall structure of the foot, but also for the arch of the foot. The cuboid, cuneiform and metatarsal bones form the transverse arch of the foot. This arch is reinforced by the important talocalcaneonavicular (or spring) ligament. The medial longitudinal arch is formed by the calcaneus, talus, navicular, cuneiforms, and medial three metatarsal bones. Finally, the lateral longitudinal arch is formed by the calcaneus, cuboid, and lateral two metatarsals bones.

Muscular Anatomy

The muscles of the foot and ankle are classified as either extrinsic muscles (originating outside the foot and ankle proper) or intrinsic muscles, originating within the foot and ankle itself. The first set of extrinsic muscles is found in the anterior compartment of the lower leg and includes the ankle dorsiflexors and toe extensors. The tibialis anterior originates from the tibia and interosseous membrane and attaches to both the medial cuneiform and first metatarsal. It is responsible for ankle dorsiflexion. Lateral to the tibialis anterior is the extensor digitorum longus that originates from the fibula and intermuscular septum and inserts on toes two through five. The extensor hallicus longus originates from the fibula and interosseus membrane and attaches to the distal phalanx of the first toe.

The next set of extrinsic muscles is found in the superficial and deep posterior compartments of the lower leg. The ankle plantarflexors are in the superficial posterior compartment. The gastrocnemius muscle is easily palpated at the posterior lower leg with its origin at the lateral and medial femoral condyles and inserting at the calcaneus via the Achilles tendon. The gastrocnemius is a secondary knee flexor and plantarflexes the foot during knee extension. The soleus is deep to the gastrocnemius in the same compartment. Its origin is at the tibia and fibula and inserts on the calcaneus. This muscle is also responsible for ankle plantarflexion. The plantaris muscle lies between these two muscles with its origin just above the knee and ends in a thin tendon at the calcaneus. The toe flexors are in the deep posterior compartment. The flexor hallucis longus (FHL) has its origin at the fibula and interosseus membrane and inserts at the first distal phalanx. Medial to the FHL is the flexor digitorum longus (FDL). Its origin is at the tibia and it inserts on the distal phalanges of toes two to five. The tibialis posterior is the most medial of the muscles. It arises from the tibia, fibula, and interosseus membrane and inserts on the navicular, cuneiform and cuboid bones and the three middle metatarsal bases. The FHL, FDL, and tibialis posterior tendons run through the tarsal tunnel, which is formed by the medial malleolus and calcaneus at its base and the flexor retinaculum as the tunnel roof.

The lateral compartment of the lower leg contains the peroneus longus and brevis muscles. These muscles are responsible for foot inversion and some ankle plantarflexion. The peroneus longus has its origin at the upper lateral fibula and inserts at the medial cuneiform and first metatarsal. The peroneus brevis origin is at the lower lateral fibula and inserts on the base of the fifth metatarsal. The intrinsic muscles of the foot are found just distal to the ankle within the plantar surface of the foot. They provide additional movement of the toes. These muscles are toe plantar flexors, toe dorsiflexors, toe abductors, and toe adductors. These muscles also act to maintain the arch of the foot. It is beyond the scope of this chapter to name them all.

PHYSICAL EXAMINATION

Table 9.1. Extrinsic Muscles of the Foot and Ankle

Muscle	Origin	Insertion	Action	Innervation
Flexor Digitorum Longus	Tibia	Distal phalanges of toes two to five	Plantarflexion of toes two to five, ankle plantarflexion, maintains foot longitudinal arch	Tibial Nerve, L5
Extensor Digitorum Longus	Fibula and intermuscular septum	Toes two to five	Dorsiflexion of toes two to five	Deep Peroneal Nerve, L5
Extensor Hallicis Longus	Fibula and interosseus membrane	First toe distal phalanx	First toe dorsiflexion	Deep Peroneal Nerve, L5
Flexor Hallicis Longus	Fibula and interosseus membrane	First toe distal phalanx	Frst toe plantarflexion, foot plantarflexion, maintains foot longitudinal arch	
Peroneal Longus and Brevis	Longus – upper lateral fibula Brevis – lower lateral fibula	Longus – Medial cuneiform and first metatarsal Brevis – 5th Metatarsal base	Foot eversion, aids plantarflexion, maintains arch	Superficial Peroneal Nerve, S1
Posterior Tibialis	Tibia, fibula, and interosseus membrane	Navicular, Cuneiform, Cuboid, and middle three metatarsal bases	Foot inversion, plantarflexion	Tibial Nerve, L5
Soleus	Tibia and fibula	Calcaneus	Foot plantarflexion	
Gastrocnemius	Lateral and medial condyles of femur	Calcaneus	Knee flexion, Foot plantarflexion	Tibial Nerve, S1, S2
Anterior Tibialis	Interosseus membrane and tibia	Medial cuneiform and first metatarsal	Ankle dorsiflexion, foot inversion	Deep Peroneal Nerve, L4, L5
Plantaris	Lateral femur	Calcaneus	Foot Plantarflexion	Tibial Nerve, S1, S2

Medical History

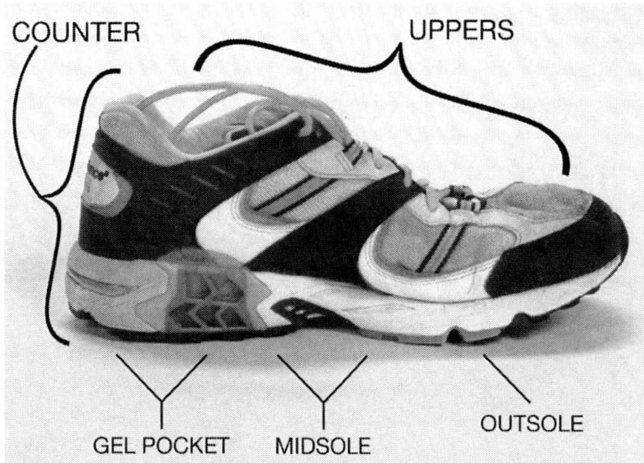

Figure 9.1. Evaluate athletic footwear for proper fit, support, and wear patterns.

In the evaluation of any orthopedic complaint, a thorough history is a critical part of your assessment. Clues from the history can suggest which focused tests or maneuvers should be used to evaluate suspected pathology. For a foot or ankle injury, questions should include those directed along the entire lower extremity as pathology at the hip or knee may play a role in the patient's current complaints.

The first question is to ascertain whether the patient has an acute or chronic injury. Acute injuries to the foot and ankle are usually caused by trauma. Ask specific questions about the nature and circumstance of the injury including the position of the foot and ankle at the time of injury, and if a "snap" or "pop" was heard or felt. Ask if there was immediate pain and swelling or if this developed over a period of time. Determine the exact location and quality of the pain, the intensity of the pain over time and what makes the pain better and worse.

In chronic foot and ankle injuries, one is often concerned about whether this is an injury that was once acute and has not healed, or whether it is due to chronic stress injury. As the foot and ankle are weight-bearing structures, they are prone to stress injury from activities that expose them to repeated stress such as running. The clinician should ascertain how much "pounding" a patient's foot and ankle receives. For example, to assess stress from running, ask how many days per week, for how many minutes, what surface is used, and what is the mileage per day and per week? You should ask about footwear, both sporting (Figure 9.1) and casual, to determine if the patient is wearing the correct shoe for his sport and his foot structure.

Finally, ask if the pain was noticed initially after the activity and then progressed to pain during the activity. This history suggests an overuse (repetitive motion) rather than acute type injury.

Observation

With foot and ankle injuries the clinician must observe the patient while he/she is ambulating. The examiner should note if the patient is using an assistive device such as crutches or a cane and describe the patient's gait, i.e., ataxic, antalgic, etc. The presence or absence of a limp should be noted as well as any ability to weight bear on the affected leg.

The patient should have both feet and ankles exposed (Figure 9.2). Shoes and socks should be removed, and the leg should be easily viewed from the knee down. Look initially for any swelling, erythema, or ecchymosis around the foot or ankle. Ensure that bony landmarks such as the medial and lateral malleolus and base of the fifth metatarsal can be easily seen. Inspect skin for lesions such as blisters, ingrown toe nails, and distal toe discolorations as they can indicate poorly fitting shoes. Careful foot examination is important for diabetic patients, as they are susceptible to infection, circulatory problems, and neuropathy in the feet. Circulation should always be assessed in this group of patients.

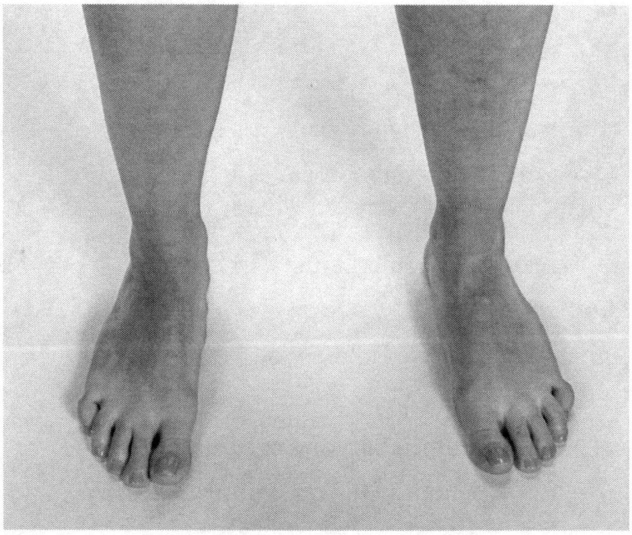

Figure 9.2. Observe feet and ankles with the patient weight-bearing.

Next, check for bony alignment. Look first at the forefoot and note any deviation of the toes. Document the presence of "hammer toes," "claw toes" and hallux valgus (bunion deformity) or varus, especially at the first MTP, as these can greatly affect ambulation. Observe the position of the forefoot in relation to the hindfoot. The forefoot can be in a straight, (rectus) position, or curved (adductus) position. The arch can be in a high (cavus) position with a rigid supinated foot, or low (planus) position with a pronated foot. The heel may be in a valgus or varus position depending on the patient's stance (Figure 9.3). The arch is best evaluated as the patient ambulates in bare feet. Evaluation of increased foot pronation with a half-squat maneuver is helpful.

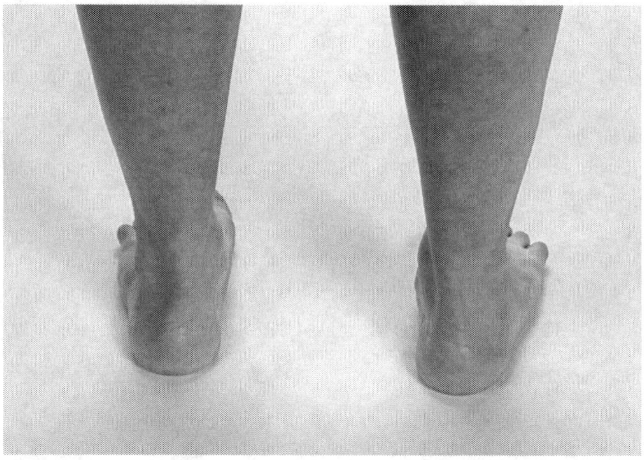

Figure 9.3. Observe heels for varus or valgus.

Palpation

Any orthopedic examination requires evaluation of both the affected and non-affected limb. The examiner should examine joints above and below the affected joint. The clinician may move from proximal to distal or vice versa; however, the examination should progress in the same way every time so that important information is not missed.

In the examination of a foot or ankle injury, begin just below the knee and palpate along the entire length of the lower leg. Be sure to palpate the proximal fibula and tibia looking for erythema, tenderness, or instability that may lead to suspicion of a syndesmotic injury. Tenderness in the area of the fibular head can indicate a Maisonneuve fracture. Follow the shafts of these bones down to the lateral and medial malleoli, respectively. Move off the lateral malleolus and palpate the anterior talofibular, calcaneofibular, and posterior talofibular ligaments

(Figure 9.4), in their order from anterior to posterior. Palpate the deltoid ligament from anterior to posterior along the medial malleolus (Figure 9.5). Then move your hands anteriorly, to check the syndesmosis, first medial to lateral and then distal to proximal. The presence of tenderness, erythema or swelling could indicate injury or "sprain" of these ligaments.

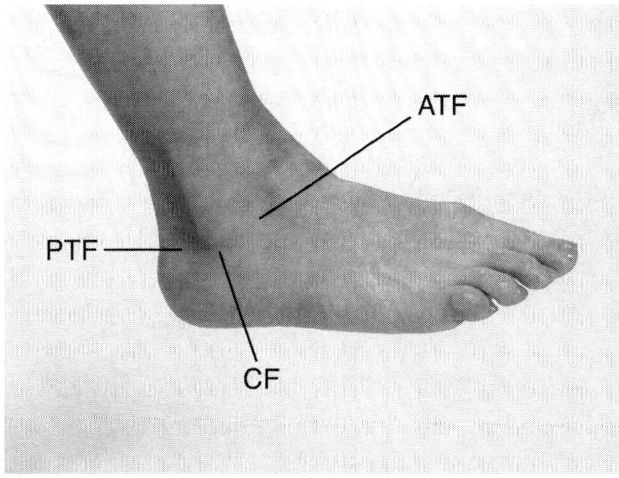

Figure 9.4. Lateral ankle ligaments.

Next, palpate the main tendons of the ankle. Check for any defects, either complete or partial, as well as masses or nodules in the Achilles tendon. Then slide your fingers along the lateral side of the ankle palpating the peroneus longus and brevis tendons. On the medial side, examine the posterior tibialis tendon. Note the presence of any tenderness, swelling or subluxation of the tendons. Be sure to also palpate the tarsal tunnel and its associated structures.

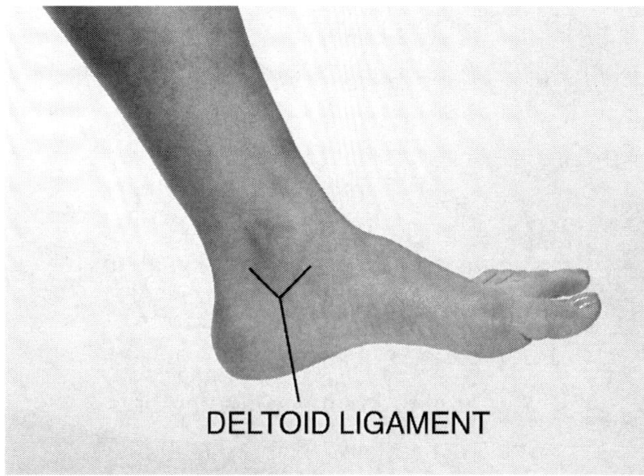

Figure 9.5. Medial Ankle ligaments.

The examiner should then palpate both the plantar and dorsal surfaces of the hindfoot and midfoot for swelling and tenderness. Important structures here include the sinus tarsi (Figure 9.6), the origin of the plantar fascia on the calcaneus, the insertion of the posterior tibialis tendon on the navicular tubercle, the calcaneocuboid and talonavicular joints, the first and second metatarsal cuneiform joints and the base of the fifth metatarsal. Fracture of this last bone, as well as damage to the peroneus brevis, can be missed if this area is not palpated. This is the most common fracture in the foot.

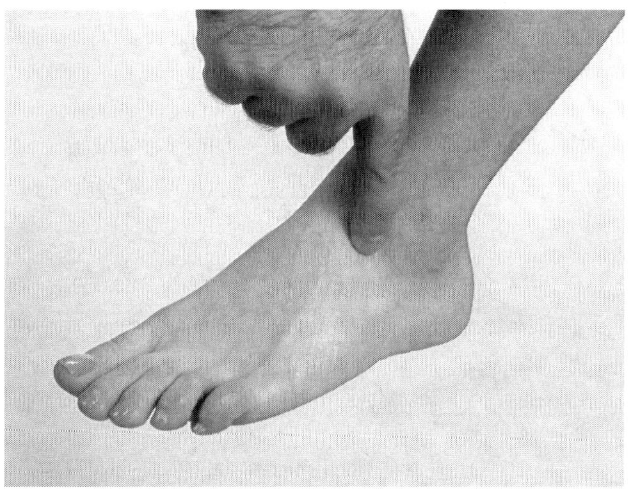
Figure 9.6. Sinus tarsi.

The final area of the foot to palpate is the forefoot. The MTP joints, especially the first MTP should be palpated. The first MTP joint can be the site of osteoarthritic change (hallux rigidus) or "turf toe" (a sprain at the first MTP joint), either of which can be debilitating. Palpate the distal and proximal interphalangeal joints looking for swelling, erythema, or deformity. Palpate the interspaces between all of the metatarsal heads, especially between the third and fourth metatarsals as pain and swelling in this area can be indicative of Morton's neuroma.

Range of Motion (ROM)

Active and passive ranges of motion of the ankle and subtalar joints should be assessed comparing the affected to the unaffected side. Range of motion should be equal bilaterally. They should be recorded in degrees. Generally accepted normal ranges of motion for the foot and ankle are as follows:

- Dorsiflexion
  - Active ROM: Patient is sitting with legs hanging off the table. Ask the patient to bring his toes up toward his nose.
  - Passive ROM: Patient sitting in same position with examiner holding tibia with one hand and examining hand moves foot into dorsiflexion (Figure 9.7). Passive normal ROM is between 15-20 degrees.
- Plantarflexion
  - Active ROM: Patient is sitting with legs hanging off the table. Ask the patient to point his toes to the floor as in pushing on a gas pedal.
  - Passive ROM: Patient sitting in same position with examiner holding tibia with one hand and examining hand moves foot into plantarflexion (Figure 9.8). Passive normal ROM is between 55-65 degrees.
- Pronation (involves both ankle and subtalar motion)
  - Active ROM: Patient is sitting with legs hanging off the table. Ask the patient to

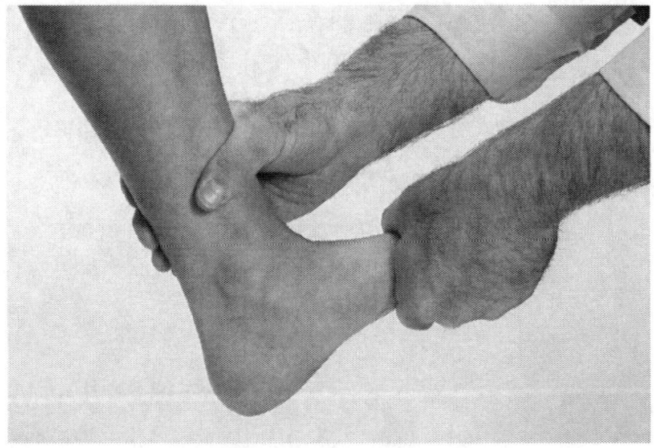

Figure 9.7. Passive dorsiflexion of the ankle.

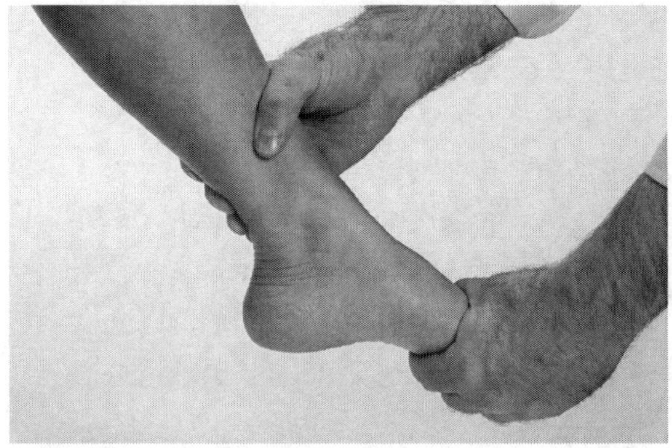

Figure 9.8. Passive plantarflexion of the ankle.

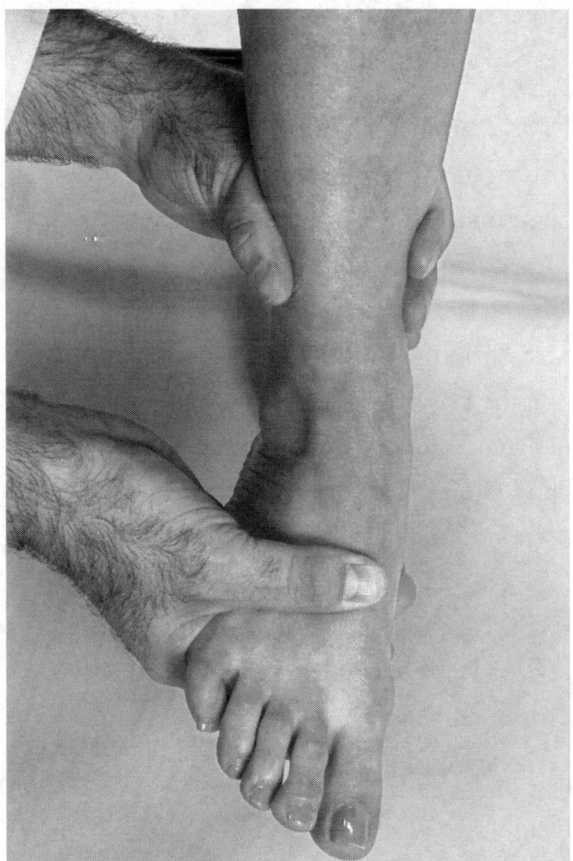

Figure 9.9. Passive pronation of the ankle.

tilt foot to the inside (eversion).

  - Passive ROM: Patient sitting in same position with examiner holding tibia with one hand and examining hand moves foot into pronation (Figure 9.9). Passive normal ROM is about 5 degrees from the neutral position.
- Supination (involves both ankle and subtalar motion)
  - Active ROM: Patient is sitting with legs hanging off the table. Ask the patient to tilt foot to the outside (inversion).
  - Passive ROM: Patient sitting in same position with examiner holding tibia with one hand and examining hand moves foot into supination (Figure 9.10). Passive normal ROM is about 20 degrees from the neutral position.

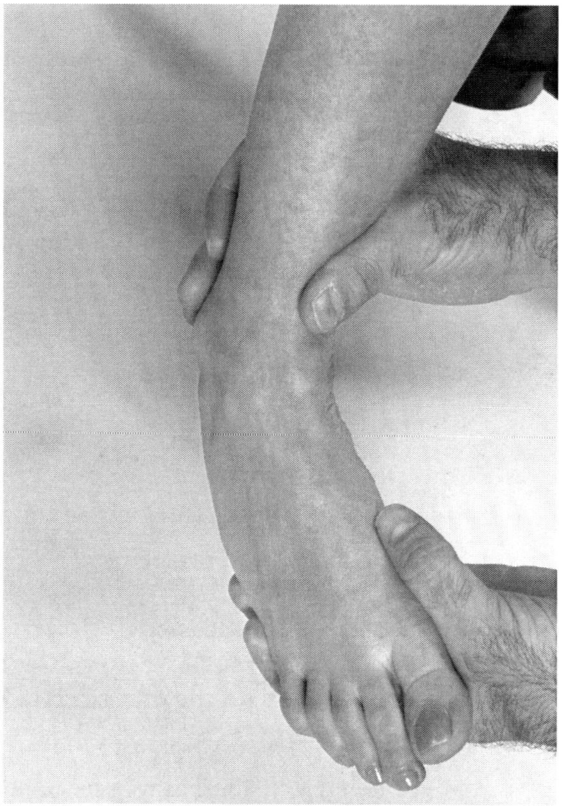

Figure 9.10. Passive supination of the ankle.

- Subtalar
  - Active ROM: Patient is lying prone with the knee flexed to 135 degrees. The patient dorsiflexes and then inverts and everts foot.
  - Passive ROM: Patient is lying prone with the knee flexed to 135 degrees. The foot is passively dorsiflexed and then inverted and everted (Figure 9.11). Passive normal ROM at the subtalar joint is between 10 and 20 degrees.

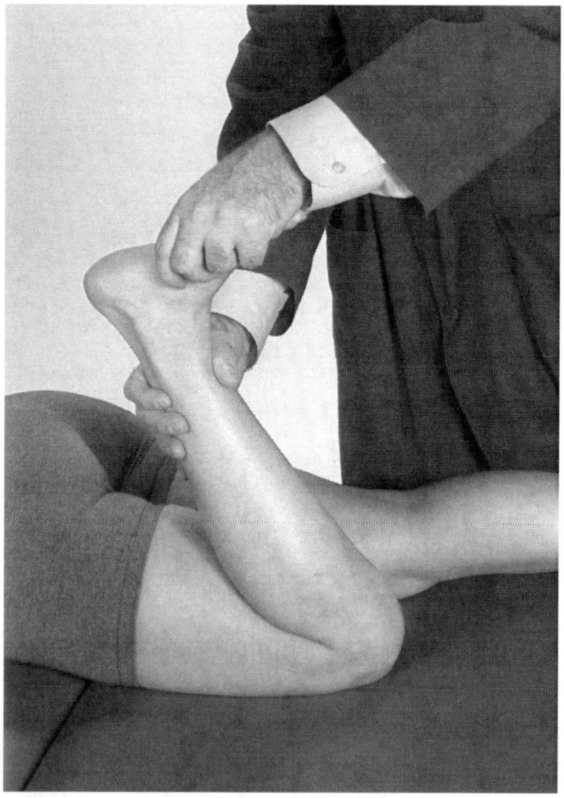

Figure 9.11. Evaluation of subtalar passive range of motion.

Neurovascular Examination

- Sensation
  - L4 Dermatome: Associated with sensation on the medial side of the ankle and foot including the medial tibia, medial malleolus and medial foot. It also includes the first MTP joint.
  - L5 Dermatome: Associated with sensation on the anterior ankle and dorsum of the foot from the first to

fourth toe.

  - S1 Dermatome: Covers the lateral foot and fifth toe dorsum.
  - Sensation can be assessed by pinprick and followed by a small brush. One can also use the two-point discrimination test previously described to test sensation.

- Reflexes
  Achilles Tendon Reflex (S1): Tested by striking Achilles tendon with reflex hammer while holding the foot in full dorsiflexion. The S1 nerve root is responsible for the Achilles tendon reflex.
- Pulses
  The important pulses in the foot and ankle region are the dorsalis pedis and posterior tibial. The dorsalis pedis is located on the dorsum of the foot near the neck of the talus. The posterior tibial pulse is found within the tarsal tunnel on the medial side of the ankle just posterior to the medial malleolus.

Manual Muscle Testing/Resisted Motion Testing

Manual muscle testing is testing of a selected muscle or muscle group against manual resistance by the examiner. This testing assesses the strength of the selected muscle or muscle group and may evoke discomfort if there is muscle or tendon injury.
The following tests should be done with the patient sitting on the edge of the exam table with legs hanging off the table. The clinician should be seated in front of the patient.

- Flexor Digitorum Longus (tibial nerve, L5): The clinician stabilizes the foot with the one hand at the calcaneus while the examining hand resists plantar flexion of toes two through five.
- Extensor Digitorum Longus (deep peroneal nerve, L5): Position is same as above but the examining hand resists dorsiflexion of toes two through five.
- Flexor Hallucis Longus (tibial nerve, L5): The clinician stabilizes the foot at the calcaneus with one hand while the examining hand resists flexion of the first MTP joint.
- Extensor Hallucis Longus (deep peroneal nerve, L5): The positioning is the same as above but the examining hand resists extension of the first MTP joint.
- Peroneus longus and brevis (superficial peroneal nerve, S1): The examiner places the foot into inversion and the patient should evert against the physician's opposite hand.
- Posterior Tibialis (tibial nerve, L5): The examiner places the foot into eversion or neutral and the patient should invert against the physician's opposite hand. Alternatively, this could be checked by having the patient "toe walk" in the office.
- Soleus (tibial nerve, S1, S2): The examiner stabilizes lower leg with one hand and patient plantarflexes against resistance by examiner.

The following tests should be done with the patient in a supine position on an examining table:

- Gastrocnemius (tibial nerve, S1, S2): The patient should be supine on examining table with knee in extension. The examiner brings the foot into dorsiflexion and the patient pushes (plantar flexes) against the resistance of the examiner's opposite hand.

- Anterior tibialis (deep peroneal nerve, L4, L5): The patient should be supine on examining table. The clinician should stabilize the lower leg while the patient dorsiflexes the foot against the resistance of the examiner's opposite hand.

PROVOCATIVE TESTS AND MANEUVERS FOR BASIC EXAM

Anterior Drawer Test. This test is performed with the patient sitting with legs hanging off the table. The stabilizing hand grasps the distal one third of the tibia and holds it in a static position. The examiner makes a "C" with his examining hand placing his four fingers around the posterior calcaneus and the examining thumb across the anterior talus. A translational force is then applied to distract the calcaneus and talus away from the stabilized lower leg in an anterior direction (Figure 9.12).

> *Positive Test*: Presence of pain or laxity in the examined ankle compared to the unaffected side.

> *Indicates*: Anterior Talofibular Ligament tear/disruption with laxity. Mild sprain with pain alone.

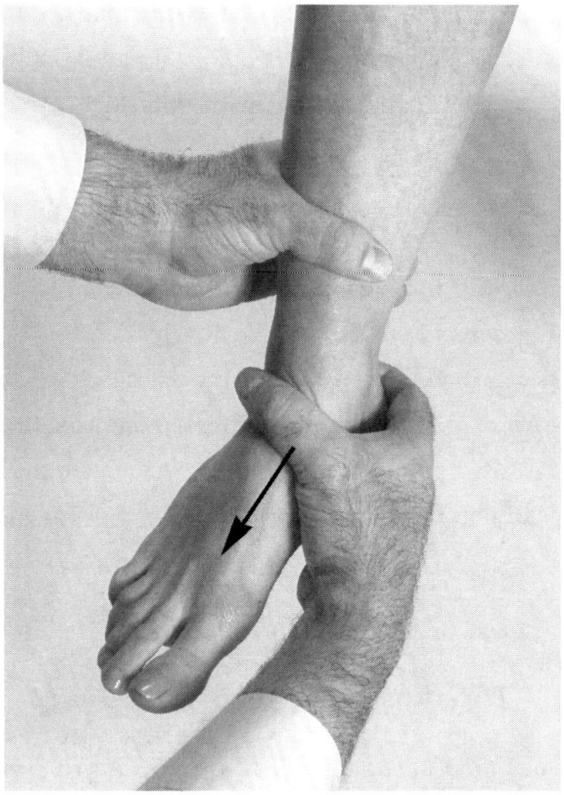

Figure 9.12. Anterior Drawer Test of the ankle.

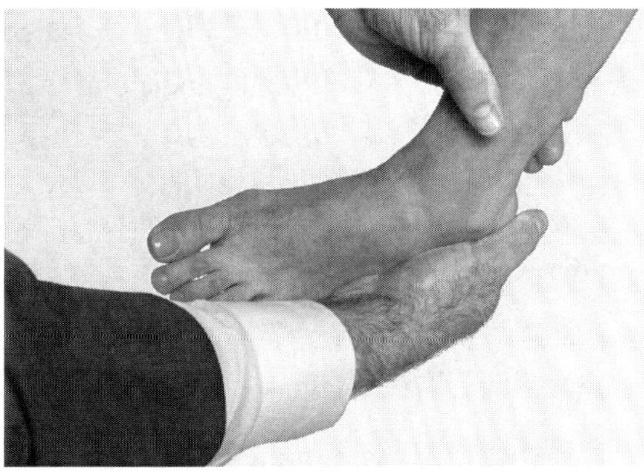

Figure 9.13. Talar Tilt Test (ankle inversion).

Talar Tilt Test. This test is performed with the patient in the same position as in the Anterior Drawer Test. The stabilizing hand of the examiner remains in the same position. The examining hand grasps either the dorsum of the foot or the inferior calcaneus and the talus is inverted to examine range of motion (Figure 9.13).

> *Positive Test:* Presence of laxity/increased range of motion (excessive tilt) or pain as compared to the unaffected side.

> *Indicates*: Anterior Talofibular and Calcaneofibular Ligament tear/disruption with laxity mild sprain with pain alone.

Eversion Test. This test is performed with the patient in the same position as in the Anterior Drawer Test. The stabilizing hand of the examiner stabilizes the lower leg. The examining hand grasps the midfoot from the plantar surface of the foot and everts the foot to examine range of motion (Figure 9.14).

Positive Test: Presence of laxity/increased range of motion or pain at end ankle ROM, as compared to the unaffected side.

Indicates: Deltoid ligament tear/disruption. Mild sprain with pain alone.

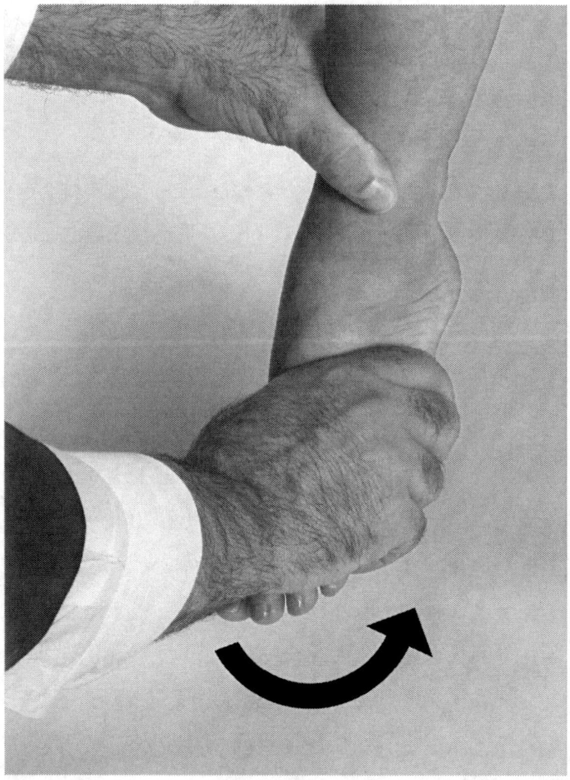

Figure 9.14. Eversion Test.

Tibiotalar Shuck Test (Cotton's Test; also known as Side-To-Side Test). This test is performed with the stabilizing hand holding the lower leg while the examining hand grasps the talus from underneath, moving it medially and laterally (Figure 9.15).

Positive Test: Production of pain and/or laxity as compared to the non-affected side.

Indicates: Syndesmosis injury/disruption.

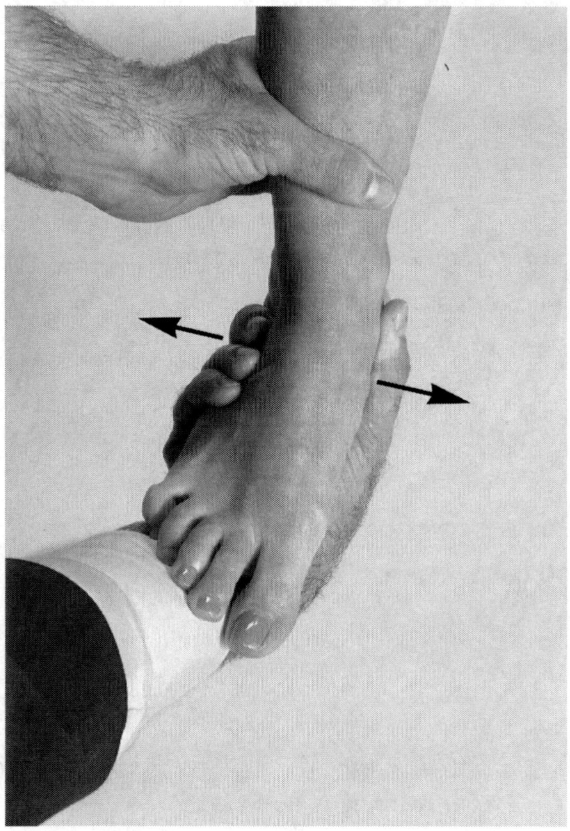

Figure 9.15. Tibiotalar Shuck Test.

Test for Calcaneocuboid Somatic Dysfunction. This test is performed with the patient prone. The clinician faces cephalad on the same side of the dysfunction. The affected foot is palpated with the thumb of the lateral hand along the plantar aspect of the cuboid.

Positive Test: Tenderness and cuboid depression on plantar surface of foot associated with decreased motion at calcaneocuboid joint.

Indicates: Excessive pronation or internal rotation of the cuboid.

Test for Navicular Somatic Dysfunction. This test is performed with the patient prone. The clinician faces cephalad on the same side of the dysfunction. The affected foot is palpated with the thumbs of both hands placed on the plantar aspect of the navicular.

Positive Test: Tenderness and medial displacement of the navicular.

Indicates: Medial displacement of the navicular.

Thompson's Test. This test is performed with the patient in a prone position with the distal 1/3 of lower leg hanging off the table. The examiner squeezes the gastrocnemius muscle and observes for plantarflexion of the ankle.

Positive Test: Absence of plantar flexion of the ankle with the maneuver.

Indicates: Rupture of the Achilles tendon.

PROVOCATIVE TESTS AND MANEUVERS FOR COMPLETE EXAM

External Rotation Test. This test is performed with the patient in the same position as the ***Talar Tilt Test.*** The stabilizing hands of the examiner remains in the same position. The examining hand externally rotates the foot against the stabilized lower leg. The talus should be included in the rotation.

Positive Test: Production of pain along the syndesmosis or medial ankle.

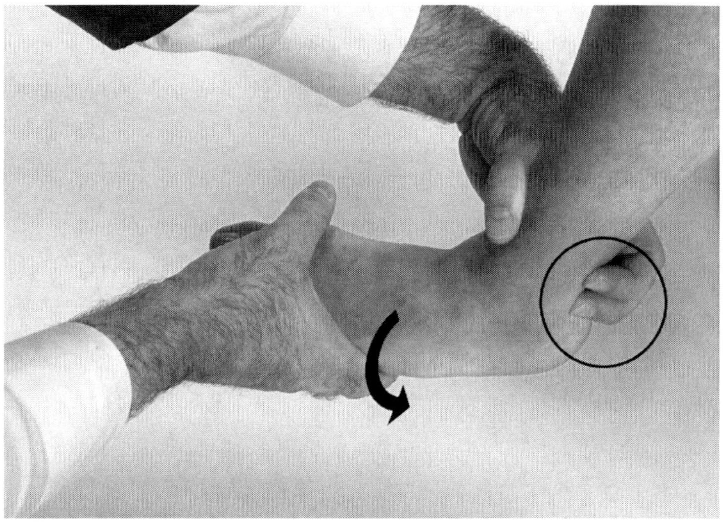

Figure 9.16. Personal Tendon Stability Test.

Indicates: Tear/disruption of the syndesmosis or the deep fibers of the medial deltoid ligament.

Peroneal Tendon Stability Test. The stabilizing hand of the examiner grasps the dorsum of the foot. The examining fingers palpate the peroneal tendons just posterior to the lateral malleolus. The foot is then passively moved to the extreme of inversion and the patient is asked to evert against resistance against the stabilizing hand, while the examining hand palpates the peroneal tendons (Figure 9.16).

Positive Test: Subluxation, catching, clicking of the tendon over the malleolus, usually associated with pain.

Indicates: Tearing of the peroneal tendon retinaculum with instability of the peroneal tendons and/or fracture of the lateral malleolus.

(Syndesmosis) Squeeze Test. The examiner places the thenar eminence of one hand against the tibial shaft and the thenar eminence of the other hand against the fibular shaft. The examiner then squeezes for 2-3 seconds followed by a brisk release (Figure 9.17).

Positive Test: Production of pain at the level of the syndesmosis.

Indicates: Syndesmosis tear/disruption.

Kleiger's Test. This test is performed with the patient seated. The knee is flexed to 90 degrees and the ankle is dorsiflexed to 90 degrees. The examiner then externally rotates the affected foot (Figure 9.18).

Positive Test: Production of pain with rotation at the level of the syndesmosis and/or mortise of the ankle.

Indicates: Syndesmosis injury/disruption.

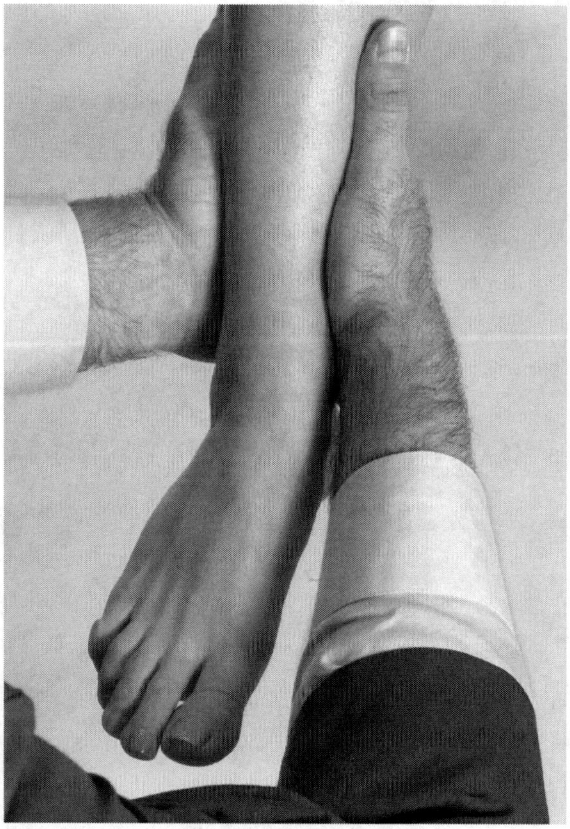

Figure 9.17. Squeeze Test.

COMMON CONDITIONS

- Fractures
  - Distal Fibula
  - Distal Tibia
  - Talar Dome
  - Talus
  - Calcaneus
  - Cuboid
  - Navicular
  - Cuneiform
  - Metatarsals (especially base of 5th)
  - Phalanges
  - Stress Fractures of any of the above bony structures
- Sprains
  - Acute Inversion Ankle Sprains (Lateral)
  - Chronic Inversion Ankle Instability (Lateral)
  - Eversion Ankle Sprains (Medial)
  - Eversion-External Rotation Ankle Sprains (Syndesmotic)

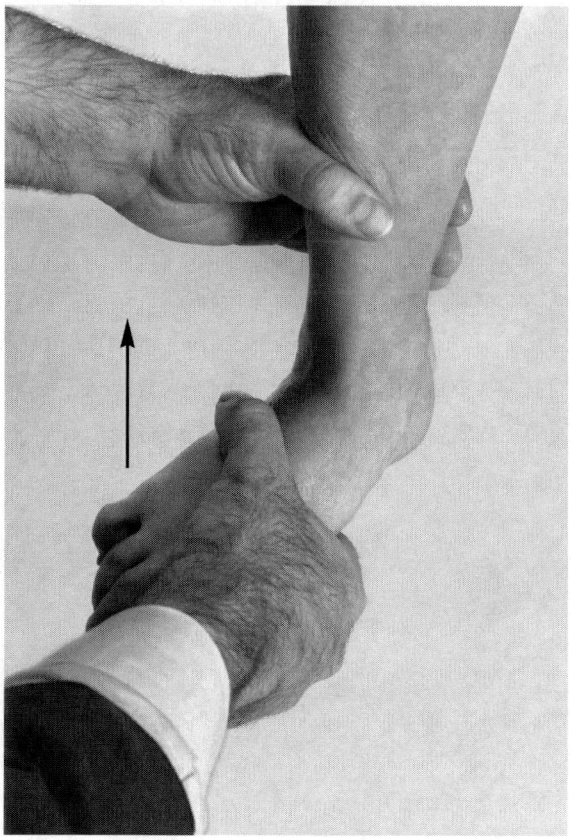

Figure 9.18. Kleiger's Test.

- Tendonitis
  - Posterior Tibialis Tendonitis
  - Flexor Hallucis Longus Tendonitis
  - Anterior Tibialis Tendonitis
  - Peroneal Longus Tendonitis
  - Peroneal Brevis Tendonitis
  - Peroneal Tendon Subluxation
  - Achilles Tendonitis
- Related Conditions of Lower Leg/Foot
  - Gastrocnemius or Achilles' Strain
  - Soleus Strain
  - Retrocalcaneal Bursitis
  - Turf Toe or Hallux Rigidus
  - Morton's Neuroma
  - Plantar Fasciitis
  - Hallux Valgus Deformity
  - Osteoarthritis
  - Tarsal Tunnel Syndrome
  - Os Trigonum Syndrome
  - Chronic Exertional Compartment Syndrome
  - Medial Tibial Stress Syndrome ("Shin Splints"/Overuse Myositis)
  - Navicular/Cuboid Somatic Dysfunction

CONDITIONS THAT SHOULD NOT BE MISSED DUE TO POSSIBLE MORBIDITY OR MORTALITY

- Fractures (See above)
  - epiphyseal (Salter-Harris)
  - fibular head (Maissoneuve)
  - Talar Dome
  - Calcaneal
  - 5th metatarsal base or body (Jones Fracture)
- Dislocations
- Acute compartment syndromes
- Tumors
- Neurologic Injury
- Acute Rupture of Achilles' Tendon
- Splitting of Peroneal Tendon
- LisFranc Sprains of foot

REFERENCES

1. Hoppenfeld S. *Physical Examination of the Spine and Extremities.* East Norwalk, CT: Appleton and Lange; 1976:197-235.
2. Karageanes SJ. *Principles of Manual Sports Medicine.* Philadelphia, PA: Lippincott Williams & Wilkins; 2005.
3. Magee DJ. *Orthopedic Physical Assessment.* Third Ed. Philadelphia, PA: W.B. Saunders Company; 1997:599-672.